CONDITION
THE NBA WAY

CONDITION
THE NBA WAY

BILL FORAN
MIAMI HEAT
Project Coordinator

ROBIN POUND
PHOENIX SUNS
Associate Coordinator

Al Biancani
SACRAMENTO KINGS

Dennis Householder
WASHINGTON BULLETS

Sol Brandys
MINNESOTA TIMBERWOLVES

Bob King
DALLAS MAVERICKS

Greg Brittenham
NEW YORK KNICKS

Bob Medina
SEATTLE SUPERSONICS

Mark Grabow
GOLDEN STATE WARRIORS

David Oliver
ORLANDO MAGIC

Roger Hinds
ATLANTA HAWKS

Chip Sigmon
CHARLOTTE HORNETS

Carl Horne
LOS ANGELES CLIPPERS

Mick Smith
PORTLAND TRAILBLAZERS

FOREWORD
LENNY WILKENS
ATLANTA HAWKS

CADELL & DAVIES
NEW YORK

Cadell & Davies™
An imprint of Multi Media Communicators, Inc.
575 Madison Avenue, Suite 1006
New York, NY 10022

Special thanks to The Management Group of the NBCCA—Joel Benson and Michael Wohl.

Drawings by Tim Ladwig.

Cover design by Jim Hellman and Tim Ladwig.

Photographers: David Phillips, Bob Rannells, and Roc Smith.

Prepress: Paul Dougan, Desktop Direct Inc. N.Y.

Library of Congress Cataloging-in-Publication Data:

Foran, Bill.
    Condition the NBA Way / Bill Foran, Robin Pound,
Bob King, Sol Brandys: foreword by Lenny Wilkens.
        p.   cm.
    ISBN 1-56977-886-8: $19.95
        1. Basketball—Training. 2. Physical education and training.
3. Physical fitness. I. Pound, Robin. II. King, Bob.
III. Brandys, Sol. IV. Title.
GV885.35.F66 1994
796.323'07—dc20   94-40803
                                                            CIP

10 9 8 7 6 5 4 3 2 1

Printed in the United States of America with thanks to Lenn Mooney and all the employees of Rose Printing who helped in the production of this book.

We would like to thank the many NBA players who permitted us to photograph them for this book and who were so generous in providing their insights on conditioning and its importance to their careers.

FOREWORD

"If you want to perform or excel at the peak of your abilities, then you must prepare yourself mentally, emotionally, and most of all physically.

"An athlete who takes the time to condition his or her body is more ready to meet the challenges of competition and, therefore, succeed at a higher rate. Everyone is aware that strength and conditioning programs have become very sophisticated today. Wise athletes will take advantage of the detailed programs described in this book."

Lenny Wilkens, Head Coach
Atlanta Hawks
NBA Coach of the Year, 1994

CONTENTS

INTRODUCTION

The sheer abundance of information available now in the strength and conditioning fields can often be confusing for young athletes and coaches.

Within the pages of this book, the top NBA strength and conditioning coaches make it all clear and understandable. We are constantly trying to be at the forefront of our field. We develop and implement total conditioning programs for the world-class athletes of the NBA on a year-round basis. With this book you will be able to utilize this same information.

This book gives you practical tools for improving yourself as a basketball player and as a well-rounded athlete.

This book has nine major sections: Warming Up, Stretching, Cooling Down; Conditioning; Agility; Plyometrics; Speed; Weight-Training; Nutrition; BC Power Rating; and Putting It All Together. Any athlete who practices the principles described in this book will learn how to run faster, jump higher, move more quickly, be stronger, carry less body fat, and reduce their chances for injury. Each of the sections are explained thoroughly with details for how you can incorporate the principles into your daily, weekly, monthly, and yearly plans.

An important feature of CONDITION THE NBA WAY is an innovative self-test—the BC (Basketball Conditioning) Power Rating™—which we created especially for this book. The BC Power Rating consists of 8 physical tests which will monitor your improvement as an athlete. Once you have obtained your first rating you can begin to monitor your progress as you work with this book, and even compare yourself to others. It is our sincere hope that you and your friends will have fun seeing who can best improve their BC Power Rating.

For the sake of ease and consistency, this book was written using male pronouns.

STEPS TO SUCCESS

The Steps to Success are key to understanding how the entire conditioning program fits together. We have included several significant ways that you can avoid frustration or failure and build success into your program.

Designing your Steps to Success is similar to creating a successful game plan in basketball. It takes teamwork. So you might ask your coach, parents, or a good friend to help you once you have read over this section.

1) **Set your goals.** CONDITION THE NBA WAY outlines a detailed conditioning plan for you. After reading the book, test yourself with the eight BC Power Rating tests.

   Short-term goals: Based on your initial BC Power Rating, write down realistic and attainable goals for each of the eight BC Power Rating tests. Then test yourself again in about a month.

   Long-term goals: Determine where you would like to be physically in one year, including your body weight, strength levels, speed levels, as well as your BC Power Rating.

   Remember, your goals need to be realistic and attainable. You may want to discuss them with your coach.

2) **Be positive.** On a regular basis, tell yourself you can attain all your goals. Being positive will help you stay motivated and committed to your total conditioning program.

3) **Get a training partner.** When two or three motivated young athletes work out together, they can inspire each other to greater levels of achievement.

4) **Execute.** Do it! Talking or thinking about how great you are going to do tomorrow doesn't get the job done, and remember: "Don't just do it, do it right." Once you have set your goals and made your commitment, start taking action.

5) **Evaluate your progress.** Re-test yourself with the BC Power Rating. See what goals you have attained and re-set your goals. You'll find that you have certain strengths and weaknesses. By addressing your weaknesses and turning them into strengths, you'll be developing yourself into a "well-rounded athlete." If you continue to follow our plan correctly, we guarantee you'll attain success.

A FINAL WORD

The exercises and drills in this book follow carefully planned guidelines. By following these guidelines closely, you will obtain the best possible results. Before beginning any new exercise program, be sure to see your physician.

Good luck with your conditioning!

Bill Foran
President, NBCCA

Warming Up, Stretching, Cooling Down

To stretch or not to stretch—that is the question. NBA players and coaches praise it. Here's what some NBA players and coaches have to say about the subject.

"For today's athletes, stretching ranks up there with increasing strength and skill level," says **Brian Hill**, Head Coach of the **Orlando Magic**. "It helps prevent the muscle tears and other nagging injuries which keep players off the court during the season."

"Stretching has improved my overall agility," says **Danny Manning** of the **Phoenix Suns**. "When I stretch before games, I feel more ready to perform, and I get into the groove easier."

"Flexibility has always been a big part of my game in high school, college, and now in my professional career," says **Hersey Hawkins** of the **Charlotte Hornets**. "The more years I put into the league, the more I realize how important stretching is."

"When I was a player, we never stretched," says **Bob Hill**, Head Coach of the **San Antonio Spurs**. "Therefore I questioned the importance of it when I became a coach. As I saw how stretching helped my team decrease ankle, hamstring, and groin injuries, I bought into the concept. Now I feel stretching and lifting not only help with maintenance during the season, but also athletes are better at the end of the season when it all counts."

The practice of stretching has evolved in the last twenty-five years from something very general to something very specialized, almost a science. Perhaps the most exciting part of this evolution is that the practice of stretching remains clear and simple. Nowadays people with all sorts of athletic and non-athletic backgrounds can practice stretching with ease and pleasure. Recently most coaches have changed their old way of thinking and now include stretching as an integral part of their conditioning regimen.

WHY STRETCHING IS IMPORTANT

The primary goal of every stretching program is to increase the range of motion (ROM) of specific joints in your body. This increase in ROM has been found to be one of the main components for improving a person's overall health and fitness.

The importance of full ROM is even more significant for athletes. Why? Because an athlete's physical well-being and performance are directly related to the ability of his muscles to move through a wide range of motions. Once an athlete begins a structured stretching program, he will be able to see and feel the rewards of increased flexibility in two vital areas:

1. INCREASED PERFORMANCE

- increased power
- increased speed
- increased muscle recovery time
- reduced muscle tension
- helps to prepare athletes both mentally and physically

2. DECREASED INJURIES

- decreased strains (muscles)
- decreased sprains (tendons)
- decreased overuse injuries
- decreased lower back spasms and/or pain
- reduced muscle soreness throughout the body

> "Being flexible prevents nagging injuries," says **Jeff Turner** of the **Orlando Magic**. "I've never had a muscle strained in my career because I've always stretched."

ANATOMY AND PHYSIOLOGY OF STRETCHING

Before you begin to take up stretching in a serious way, you need to understand a few things about how your body is constructed (anatomy) and how the body works (physiology). A basic knowledge of the human anatomy is very important to athletes. It helps them understand why muscles are stretched in certain ways and why they're not stretched in others (see appendix for diagrams). In particular, you should learn a few things about joints, bones, cartilage, and ligaments.

The human body has a fascinating system of movement. All movement in our bodies revolves around our joints. The ROM of joints can either limit or promote your body's ability to move efficiently.

As mentioned earlier, by increasing your ROM, you will directly increase your capacity to move and perform basketball skills.

At the same time, increasing your ROM means that you will actually decrease the chances for injuring your joints. The most effective way you can promote increased joint flexibility, or ROM, is by regularly performing the stretching exercises you will learn in this chapter.

To help you understand how joints move, look at how your joints are structured. A typical joint is composed of muscles, tendons, bones, cartilage, and ligaments. Tendons connect muscle to bone, forming what is called the "musculotendinous" unit.

The amazing thing about muscles is that they are elastic, or like a rubber band; they have the ability to stretch. Muscles also can contract or shorten. Because of their unique ability to stretch and contract, muscles allow a great range of motion in the joints.

Bones and cartilage provide structural support and joint surfaces in order to permit movement to occur more easily. Ligaments are the primary stabilizing tissues for bones. Ligaments connect bones to bones.

> "I have to stretch before each practice and before each and every game," says **Del Curry** of the **Charlotte Hornets**. "I can tell a big difference in how I feel and perform. I'll also stretch a lot during the off-season, before and after training to help prevent injury."

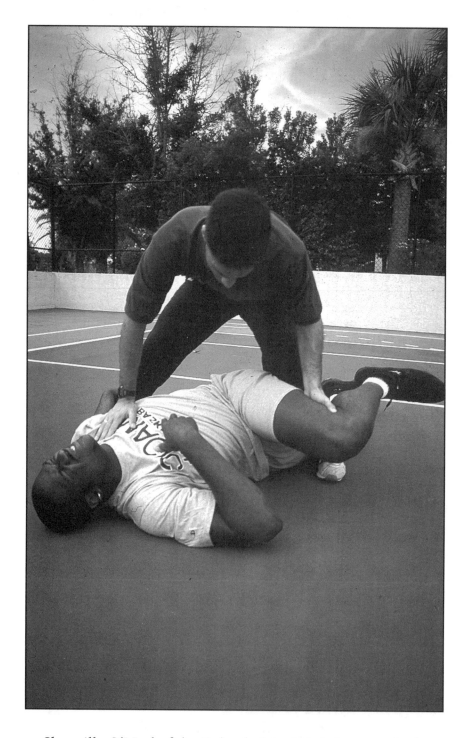

Shaquille O'Neal of the **Orlando Magic** is being stretched by his strength and conditioning coach **David Oliver.**

QUESTIONS & ANSWERS ABOUT STRETCHING AND FLEXIBILITY

1. Is breathing during stretching exercises important?

Definitely. You should breath slowly and rhythmically during all stretching. Your muscles need oxygen. Exhale as you bend forward and then breathe slowly as you hold the stretch. If a stretch inhibits your natural breathing pattern, ease up on the stretch so that you can breathe naturally.

2. What about the popular saying, "No pain, no gain"?

You should never continue an exercise if you are experiencing pain. Pain is your body's way of telling you to stop. While stretching you should feel tension, not pain or discomfort.

3. Why do people become less flexible and sustain injuries?

The rapid growth in adolescence causes muscles and bones to grow very fast. This places a great amount of stress on the joints. They become tight and pull on the bones in an irregular manner causing joint problems to occur. Unless a person stretches regularly, his muscles won't have a chance to maintain their flexibility.

As people age, joints lose their range of motion in direct response to decreased physical activity. In turn, joints experience pain and their range of motion decreases even more. This trend continues unless a person does something about it.

MUSCLE PROPERTIES

Two basic properties of a muscle are:

1. It can shorten or contract; and
2. It can lengthen or stretch.

These two basic movements maintain a close working relationship. In fact, all movement in your body depends on this relationship!

How can this possibly be? The reason is that whenever a muscle shortens/contracts, there is at the same time an immediate lengthening/stretching of the opposite muscle group. For example, when performing a free throw, the triceps muscle group contracts during the follow-through while the biceps muscle group lengthens, allowing for full extension at the elbow joint.

As you can imagine, you can greatly enhance your ability to perform when you condition your muscles so that they can perform at their optimum level.

As mentioned earlier, muscles are attached to bones by tendons. They are usually, though not always, attached in two places. A basic knowledge of the human anatomy is important in the athlete's understanding of why muscles are stretched in different ways. A more in-depth understanding of muscle anatomy is vital for those coaches performing passive stretching on their players.

WHAT MAKES A MUSCLE WORK

Muscles are made up of muscle fibers. Muscle fibers have both elastic and contractile properties, which work closely together to control movement. At a microscopic level, muscle fibers possess nerve receptors. These are so sensitive that they can sense stretching and tension developed in your muscles. These two receptors are called muscle spindles and golgi tendon organs (GTO). These are commonly referred to as proprioceptors. They act as stretch and tension receptors and are responsible for regulating your balance and helping you handle spatial relationships.

Muscle spindles run parallel to muscle fibers while golgi tendon organs are located at the junction where muscles and tendons meet. Muscle spindles respond to both the rate and length of stretch. Golgi tendon organs sense muscle tension.

MUSCLE SAFETY MECHANISM

The built-in safety mechanism that protects your body against extreme ranges of motion is called the myotatic stretch reflex.

When muscle spindles are rapidly stretched, they elicit a reflex response that activates a contraction in the same muscle. Thus, they resist any more lengthening, protecting against potential muscle strains. Always listen to your body. Stop stretching if you experience any pain or discomfort.

If the rate of stretch is rapid, this safety mechanism will protect the muscle from overstretching by initiating a forceful contraction. This built-in safety mechanism is the primary reason we employ static stretching (holding a stretch) over ballistic stretching (bouncing). This also explains how ballistic stretching activates this reflex and actually tightens the muscles that are being stretched. Basically, when you stretch too far or too quickly you tighten the muscle you are trying to stretch.

CONDITIONING TIP: When a muscle is stretched rapidly, that same stretch will elicit a forceful and rapid muscle contraction. Do not bounce! Bouncing will cause more harm than good.

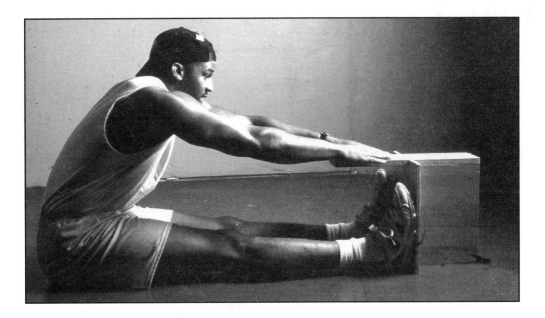

Labradford Smith of the **Sacramento Kings** is checking the flexibility of his hamstrings and lower back with a sit and reach test.

WARM-UP

There are two phases of a warm-up.

General warm-up is usually the earliest portion of the warm-up process. During this phase an athlete will elevate his body core temperature by performing physical activities such as light jogging, easy rope jumping or calisthenic-type exercises. These activities should be performed for 5 to 10 minutes or until sweating begins. Following these general exercises, the athlete should perform a stretching program to include all major muscle groups.

Once the athlete completes the full-body stretching routine (10 to 12 minutes), he can move into the *specific warm-up*, which involves activities that are more specific to the sport. Specific warm-ups include dynamic stretching, form running (multi-directional), and the standing drills outlined in the next few pages.

The warm-up process should take approximately 20 minutes and should prepare the athlete for the more physical demands to follow. The passive and dynamic stretching programs should prepare muscles to move through their fullest range of motion.

Here is an example of what a typical warm-up program should look like.

GENERAL WARM-UP

Jogging (forward, back, shuffle, carioca):   3 minutes

Jumping rope:
   double leg
   right leg
   left leg   5 minutes
   double leg

PASSIVE STRETCH (STATIC)

Full body stretch   12 minutes

SPECIFIC WARM-UP—DYNAMIC STRETCHING

Standing drills:

kick-through left	2 sets of 15 repetitions
kick-through right	2 sets of 15 repetitions

Movement drills:

marching	2 sets of 20 yards
high knee skipping	2 sets of 20 yards
heel kicks	2 sets of 20 yards
backward running	2 sets of 20 yards
forward strides	2 sets of 20 yards

} 5 to 7 minutes

COOL-DOWN

Much as the warm-up prepares you for physical exertion, cool-down is vital for enhancing muscle recovery and returning the body to its resting state.

After vigorous activity it's very important to bring the body back to its resting state slowly. Cooling down usually involves a session of easier exercise like light jogging or other physical activity for 5 to 10 minutes following workouts. Stretching of the lower back, hamstrings, quadriceps, along with any other muscle groups you choose is also appropriate.

Many teams in the NBA use these cool-down sessions as a part of their daily routines. There are two main reasons for this.

1. Continued circulation provided by the cooling-down process allows the body to restore proper fluid, electrolyte, enzyme, and nutrient balance in the muscle cells. This helps muscles recover faster and may reduce the potential for muscle cramping and injuries during future workouts. This would be especially true during two-a-day sessions.

2. The energy reserves (ATP and CP) of your muscles are brought back to their normal resting levels. Continued circulation provided by the cool-down brings new oxygen to the lungs, blood, and muscles. This helps to break down the acids found in the blood and working muscles that were created by the vigorous activity. One metabolic acid you may have heard of is lactate or lactic acid. Your cool-down helps convert lactic acid back to glucose.

It's well documented that sports like basketball, which are anaerobic in nature produce lactate in blood and muscle as a product of the high-intensity work. So it's in your best interest to do what the pros do; that is, stay healthy by performing both a warm-up and a cool-down.

Here is a review of what the cool-down may look like.

- Light jog   3 minutes
- Abdominal work   3 minutes
- Free-throw shooting   5 to 10 minutes
- Stretching   5 to 10 minutes

This is only one example. Coaches may design cool-downs that work better for their teams.

CONDITIONING TIP: Stretching is usually very effective following practice because muscles are warm and are capable of greater ranges of movement. This does not mean that stretching before practice should be omitted. To avoid risk of injury always stretch before and after a workout.

Proper warm-up is essential in preparing an athlete for practice or competition. Every warm-up session should include a stretching portion with both static and dynamic stretching. There are four different stretching techniques that will be discussed in this section of the chapter. They include:

1. Static stretching (individual stretching)
2. Dynamic stretching
3. Passive stretching (facilitated or partner stretching)
4. PNF (Proprioceptive neuromuscular facilitation)

ORDER OF STRETCHING

It is important to understand that the order in which you stretch should be considered. It is a common practice that a stretching program starts with center of movement stretches. That is the back and hips followed by the hamstrings. The reason being, in order to facilitate the maximum potential for full body flexibility one must first stretch the muscles which effect the rest of the body. Most movement is generated through your center of gravity (lower back and hips). Your hips and lower back are directly influenced by the hamstring muscle group. Following these stretches perform groin (adductor), quadriceps, and then periphery (shoulders, arms, hands, calf, ankles, feet) stretches.

Stretching the largest muscle groups first allows for greater potential flexibility in the smaller muscle groups. So, to repeat, the order is:

Back (torso)
Hips (pelvic region)
Hamstrings
Groin (adductors)
Quadriceps (calf, ankles, feet)
Shoulders, arms, wrist, hands
Neck

This is a general guideline. There are occasions when time constraints or certain situations force you to change the order. Just remember that stretching larger muscle groups first will usually be the most appropriate way.

THE STRETCHING PROGRAMS

Every warm-up session should contain a stretching portion comprised of both static and dynamic stretching.

INDIVIDUAL STATIC STRETCHING

Static stretches are those that are held in a fixed range of motion for a given period of time. You should move into all static stretches slowly until a good feeling develops. That is to say, you may feel some discomfort, but you should never feel pain.

Here are some guidelines to follow when performing your static stretching: hold each stretch 15 to 20 seconds; repeat each movement twice; stretch 5 to 7 times each week; and always try to do a full body stretch.

STANDING STRADDLE, RIGHT LEG

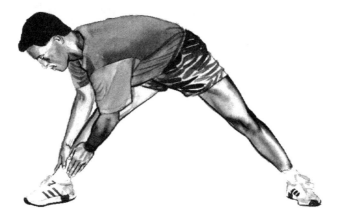

- Perform standing in a straddle position.
- Keep knees slightly bent and toes pointed outward at a 45° angle.
- Slowly bend from the waist, bringing your chest toward your knee.
- Keep your back flat.
- Stretch until you feel tension in your hamstrings.

Hold 15 seconds
Repeat twice

MUSCLES STRETCHED: hamstrings, gluteals, and erector spinae

Standing Straddle, center

- Stand in a straddle position.
- Knees slightly bent and toes pointed outward at a 45° angle.
- Bend forward from the waist, bringing your hands toward the floor in front of you.
- Keep your back flat.
- Stretch until you feel tension in your hamstrings.

Hold 15 seconds
Repeat twice

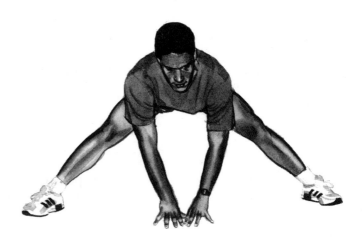

Muscles stretched: hamstrings, gluteals, erector spinae and thigh adductors

Standing Straddle, left leg

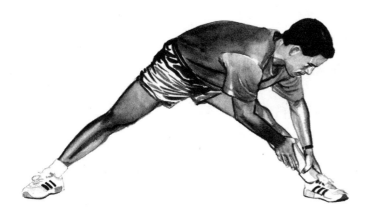

- Perform standing in a straddle position.
- Knees slightly bent and toes pointed outward at a 45° angle.
- Slowly bend from the waist, bringing your chest toward your knee.
- Keep your back flat.
- Stretch until you feel tension in your hamstrings.

Hold 15 seconds
Repeat twice

Muscles stretched: hamstrings, gluteals, and erector spinae

Side Lunge

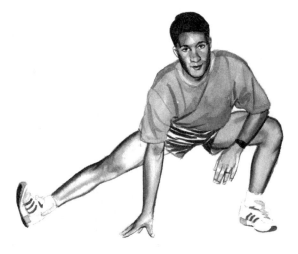

- Start in a standing straddle position.

- Facing forward, slowly lunge to the left.

- Keep your back in a straight position and your feet at a 45° angle.

- Do not let your left knee move beyond your left foot.

- Point the opposite toes up toward the ceiling (into a dorsi-flexed, heel down toe up position).

Hold 15 seconds
Repeat twice

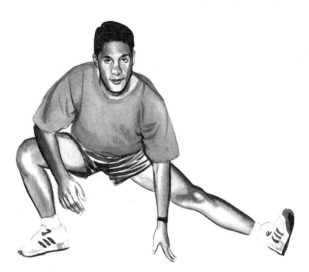

- Switch legs, repeat stretch

Muscles stretched: thigh adductors (groin) and hamstring

ILIOTIBIAL BAND STRETCH

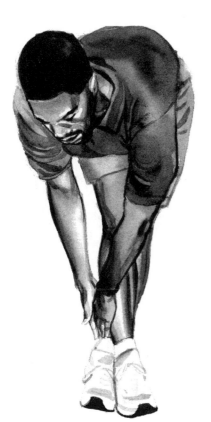

- Start in a standing position.
- Cross your right leg over your left leg.
- Keep your knees slightly bent.
- Slowly bend, moving your hands toward the ankle of your back leg.

Hold 15 seconds
Repeat twice

- Switch legs, repeat stretch.

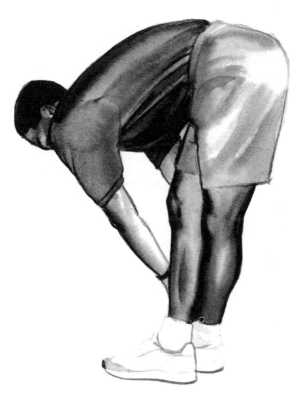

Remember to breathe, and no bouncing!

MUSCLES STRETCHED: tensor fasciae latae, gluteals, erector spinae

SEATED GROIN STRETCH

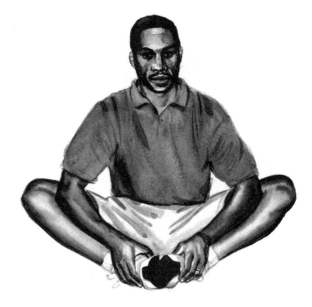

- Sit up tall in a butterfly position.
- Press your knees toward the floor with your elbows.
- Stretch until you feel tension in the inner thigh (groin).

Hold 15 seconds
Repeat twice

MUSCLES STRETCHED: thigh adductors (groin)

SUPINE GLUTEAL STRETCH

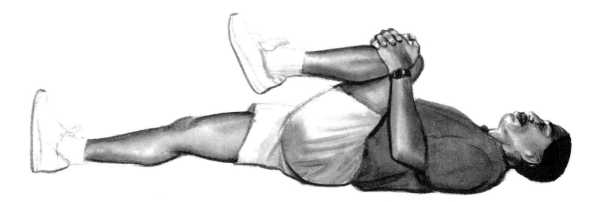

- Lie on your back.
- Keep the uninvolved knee slightly bent; you may place a towel roll under your knee.
- Slowly pull your other knee toward your chest until you feel a good stretch.

Hold 15 seconds
Repeat twice

MUSCLES STRETCHED: gluteals, erector spinae

SUPINE HAMSTRING STRETCH

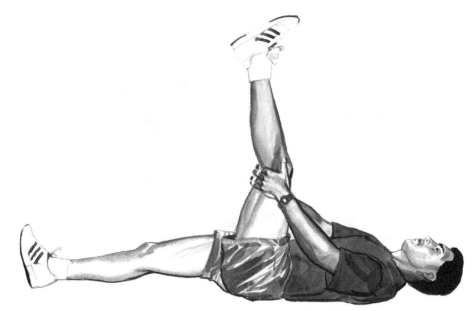

- Lie on your back.

- From supine gluteal stretch, slowly extend your leg.

- Point your toes (plantar flex).

Hold 10 seconds

- Dorsi-flex (pointing your toes toward your head).

Hold for another 10 seconds (by now you're holding for a total of 20 seconds)
Repeat twice

MUSCLES STRETCHED: hamstrings, gastrocnemius (calves) and some gluteals, depending on range of motion

CONDITIONING TIP: Don't hold your breath. As you count, say the numbers out loud—that way you will remember to breathe.

CROSSOVER STRETCH

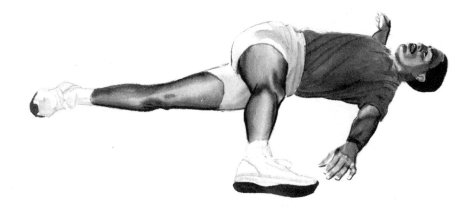

- From supine hamstring position, slowly cross your leg over and try to maintain a 90° position.
- Bring your foot toward your hand.
- Make sure to keep your shoulders flat on the floor during the stretch.

Hold 15 seconds

- Switch legs.

Repeat exercise twice

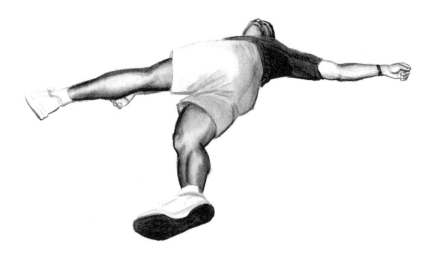

MUSCLES STRETCHED: gluteals, tensor fasciae latae, external obliques, abdominals, erector spinae

PIRIFORMIS STRETCH (DEEP LATERAL HIP)

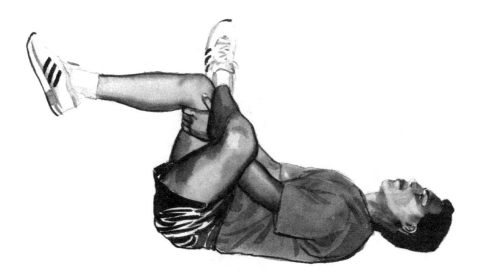

- Lying on your back, cross your left leg over your right knee.
- The ankle of your left leg should touch the right knee.
- Keep your back, shoulders, and head on the floor.
- Grab your right leg and pull it slowly, until you feel your left hip being stretched.

Hold 15 seconds
- Switch legs.
Repeat exercise twice

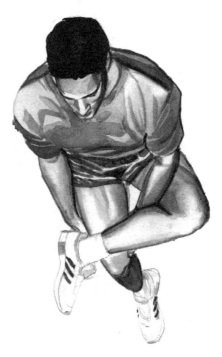

MUSCLES STRETCHED: piriformis (deep lateral hip), gluteals, tensor fasciae latae

PRETZEL STRETCH

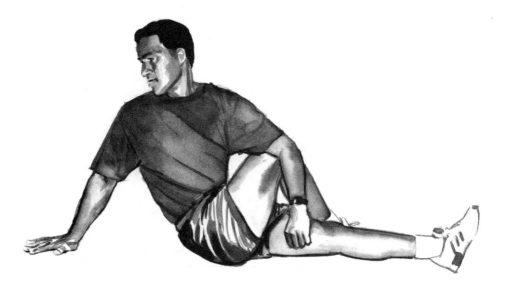

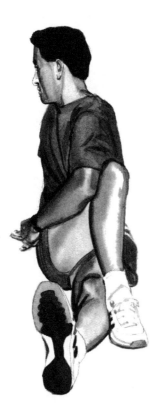

- Sitting upright, place your right hand behind you and rotate your head and shoulders toward your hand.

- Keep your left leg straight.

- Bend your right leg and cross it over your left. Push your right knee across your body with your left elbow until you feel the stretch in your right hip and torso.

Hold 15 seconds

- Switch legs.

Repeat exercise twice

MUSCLES STRETCHED: erector spinae, gluteals, abdominals

FORWARD LUNGE

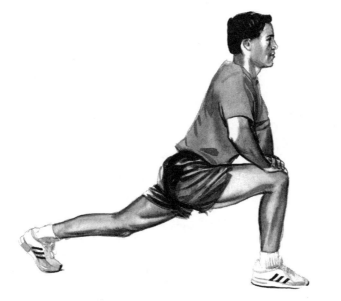

- In a standing position, lunge forward by placing your right foot forward.

- Make sure your knee does not move beyond the ball of your foot.

- Push the hip of your straight leg forward.

Hold 15 seconds

- Switch legs.

Repeat exercise twice

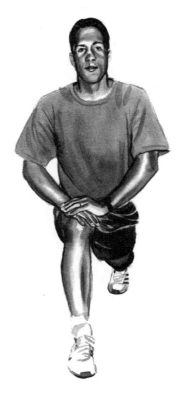

MUSCLES STRETCHED: iliopsoas, rectus femoris

STANDING QUADRICEPS STRETCH

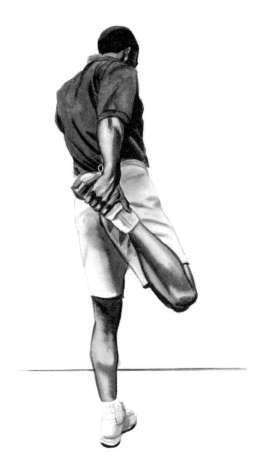

- In a standing position, balance yourself by holding on to a wall or chair.
- Grasp your right foot near the toes and pull your heel toward your gluteal muscles.
- Push your right hip forward for a better hip flexor stretch.

Hold 15 seconds

- Switch legs.

Repeat exercise twice

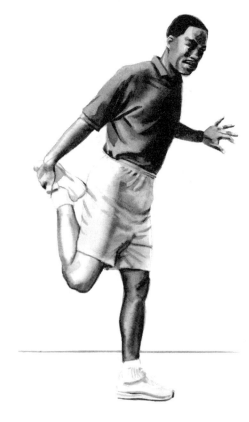

To increase flexibility hold the stretch longer. Remember never bounce.

MUSCLES STRETCHED: quadriceps, iliopsoas, anterior tibialis

STANDING CALF STRETCH

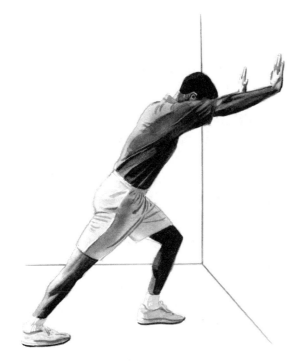

- In a standing, forward lunging position, place your hands ahead of you on a wall and support yourself.

- Press the heel of your back leg toward the floor while keeping your leg straight.

Hold 15 seconds

- Repeat with the knee slightly bent.

Hold 15 seconds

- Switch legs.

Repeat exercise twice

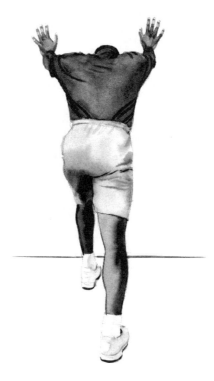

Be sure to stretch calves with legs straight as well as knees bent.

MUSCLES STRETCHED: straight leg: gastrocnemius; bent leg: soleus

DYNAMIC STRETCHING

Dynamic stretches are performed through a fuller range of motion and are more aggressive. They should be performed following static stretches, and are used to prepare you for practice or competition. Dynamic stretching helps stimulate the activity of the nervous system in specific joints.

Basically, you're letting your muscles and joints know that you are warming them up in preparation for a more vigorous activity, such as practice or competition.

Please note that dynamic stretching has also been referred to as ballistic stretching. We feel the term "dynamic stretching" better classifies this group of stretches. The term "ballistic stretching" implies bouncing. As already mentioned, bouncing movements tend to do more harm than good.

"Dynamic stretching" better describes the true nature of this form of stretching. The goal here is to increase ROM by performing a sport-specific range of motion activities. Dynamic stretching is a transitional phase between static stretches and competition. Even though dynamic stretching may not fit into the most rigid definition of "stretching"; it is extremely beneficial during warm-ups since it continues to increase a player's ROM.

There are two forms of dynamic stretching. The following pages show standing drills and sport-specific speed and movement drills.

STANDING DRILLS

SIDE TO SIDE KICK THROUGH

- Facing a wall, or holding onto a rail or fence, position your body so that you are 2 to 3 feet from the wall.

- Keep your knee slightly bent.

- Swing your right leg to the side.

- Swing your right leg across the left while swiveling your hips.

- Kick your right leg to a position where you feel a stretch in your hamstring and follow the path of the foot with your head.

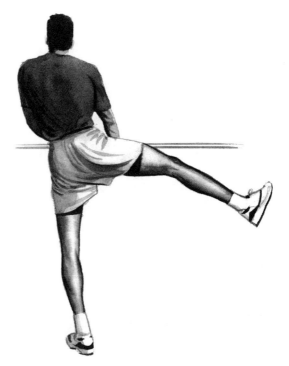

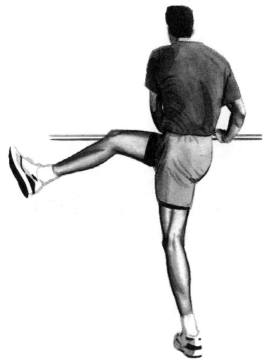

Do 10 kicks
- Switch legs, repeat exercise.

If you feel discomfort, reduce the height of the stretch.

FORWARD TO BACK KICK-THROUGH

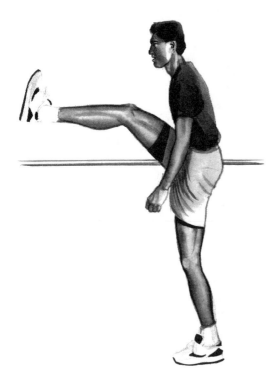

- With your right shoulder perpendicular to a wall or fence, support yourself by placing your right hand on the wall.

- Keep the knee slightly bent and maintain good posture in the back.

- Do not arch or curl your back.

- Balancing yourself with your right hand and left foot, swing your right leg up so that it is close to parallel with the floor.

- Follow the forward movement with a controlled swing backward.

- Start with easy swings, and increase the height and speed of each movement as you feel more comfortable.

Do 10 kicks with each leg
Repeat exercise

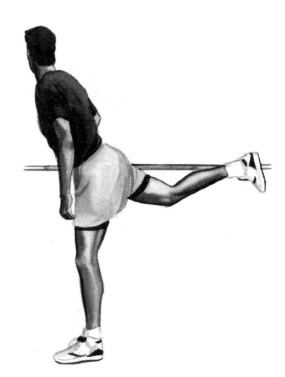

SPORT-SPECIFIC SPEED/MOVEMENT DRILLS

ANKLE FLIPS

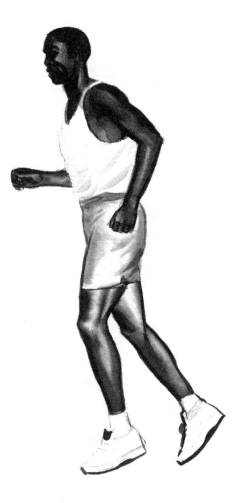

- Forcefully plantar-flex your right foot and left foot in an alternative fashion.

- Keep your knees slightly bent.

- As the right foot pushes off, the left foot should slide along the floor surface (foot is plantar-flexed with toe pointed down).

- Be sure to land on your toes and not flat-footed.

Move briskly 10 to 15 yards
Repeat

HIGH KNEE MARCHING

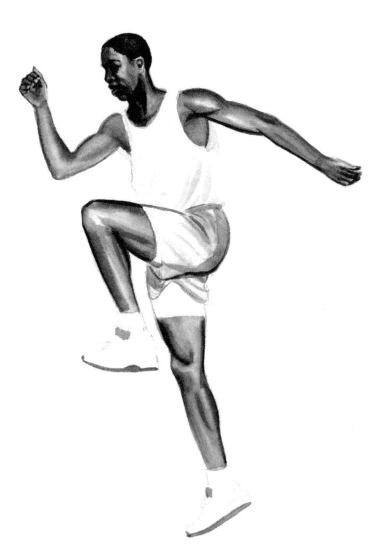

- Drive the right and left knees upward toward the chest in an alternating fashion.

- Use aggressive arm movements. Bend the arm of the straight leg, swing the opposite arm behind you. (For a further discussion of "arm movement," see the Speed chapter.)

- As you march keep the raised foot dorsi-flexed (heel down, toe-flexed upward position).

March 10 to 30 yards
Repeat

HIGH KNEE WITH LEG REACH

- Drive the right and left knees upward toward the chest in an alternating manner.
- When the knee is in the up position, extend the leg.
- With the right leg extended, finish the movement by aggressively extending the leg downward at the hip.
- Follow this movement with the opposite leg.

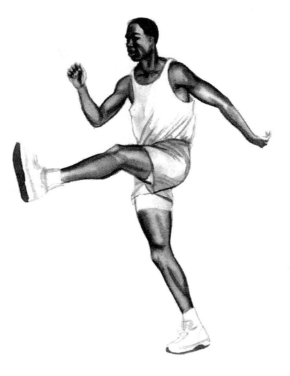

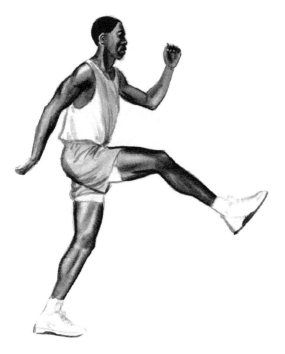

March 20 to 30 yards
Repeat

HEEL KICKS

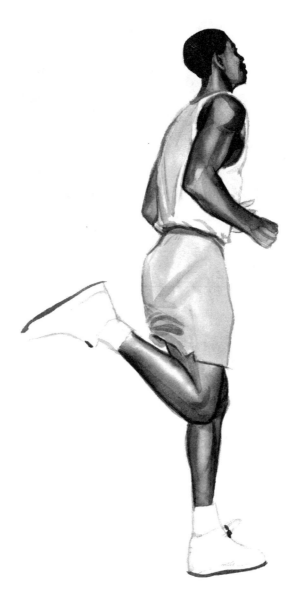

- While running forward aggressively, flex your knees.

- Try to touch your gluteals with your heels.

- The thigh should remain perpendicular to the running surface. The toes should be pointed as the heel moves toward the gluteals.

Move forward 20 yards
Repeat

CARIOCA

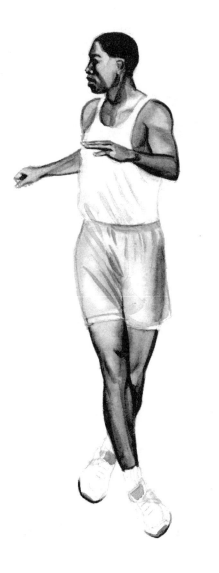

- Moving laterally, swivel your hips so that your right leg crosses in front of the left.
- Step to the side with left leg.
- Right leg crosses behind left leg.

Quickly move 30 yards
Repeat

- Switch direction, lead with opposite leg.

Repeat exercise

BACKWARD STRIDE

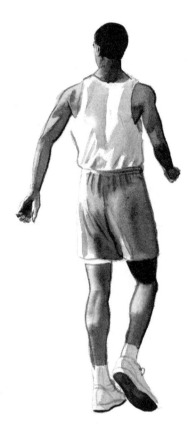

- Run backward by alternately reaching back with each foot.
- You should have an extended stride.

Run 30 yards
Repeat

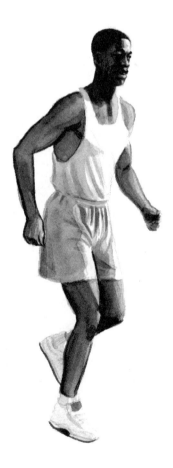

PASSIVE PARTNER STRETCHING

Passive stretching is performed on an athlete when he is being stretched by a partner or a coach. Proper technique is crucial to insure safety. Passive stretching is extremely effective in gaining increased joint range of motion. Caution should be used by the partner or coach. Injury can occur if proper care is not used.

NBA strength and conditioning coaches encourage the partner stretch. It is useful for the following reasons:

1. With partner-stretching, there's a greater chance for increased range of motion. This is due to the ability of the partner to isolate the muscle being stretched.

2. Partner-stretching helps the player to develop a personal sense of stretching by knowing what is too much of a stretch, or too little of a stretch, while stretching his teammate.

3. Partner-stretching allows for the players to interact with each other during the warm-up.

4. Partner-stretching allows the coach hands-on work with the athlete.

During the stretching phase of the warm-up, begin the partner-stretch program with lower-back (torso) and hamstring stretches. The following pages show a partner-stretch program.

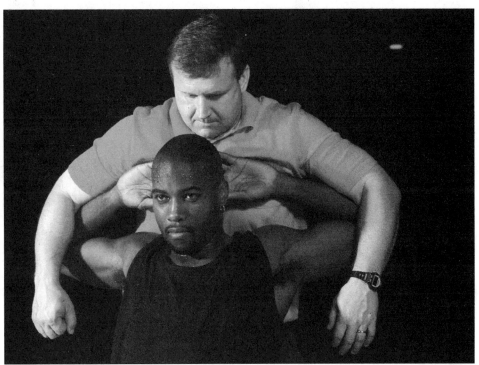

Glen Rice of the **Miami Heat** is having his chest stretched
by his strength and conditioning coach **Bill Foran.**

SEATED STRADDLE

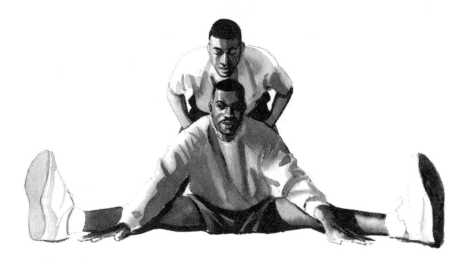

- Player sits in a straddle position (V-sit).

- Partner applies pressure—slowly and evenly—with his hands to the player's lower-mid back.

- Player should bend from the hips, keeping his back flat.

- This stretch should be performed to the right, middle, and left sides.

MUSCLES STRETCHED: hamstrings, thigh adductors, gluteals, erector spinae

DOUBLE KNEE TO CHEST

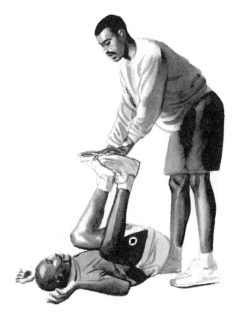

- Player lies on his back with both knees bent.

- Partner places hands on hamstrings or bottom of feet and applies pressure downward to take knees into chest.

Perform for 20 seconds
Repeat

MUSCLES STRETCHED: gluteals, erector spinae

SINGLE KNEE TO CHEST

- Player lies on his back with one knee bent with the foot raised.
- The partner presses the bottom of the player's foot toward his hip, bringing his knee to his chest.
- Partner places one hand at the bottom of his foot and the other on the knee bent.

Perform for 20 seconds.

Repeat on opposite side

Repeat exercise

MUSCLES STRETCHED: gluteals, erector spinae

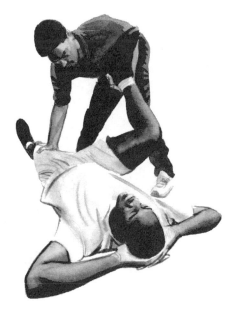

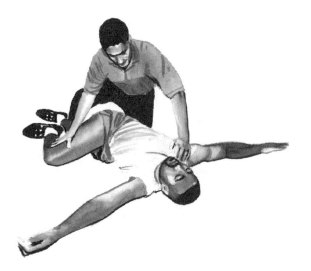

KNEE ACROSS BODY

- Go directly into this stretch by taking the raised single knee to the chest across the opposite side of the body, keeping both shoulder blades on the floor.

Perform twice, 20 seconds each knee

Repeat Single Knee to Chest and Knee Across Body stretches with the other leg

MUSCLES STRETCHED: gluteals, tensor fasciae latae, abdominals, erector spinae

LYING HAMSTRING STRETCH

- Player lies on the floor.

- While the left leg is straight, partner takes right heel of player and elevates leg to stretch hamstring.

Perform twice, holding each time for 20 seconds
Repeat on the other leg

MUSCLES STRETCHED: hamstrings, gastrocnemius (calves) and some gluteals, depending on range of motion

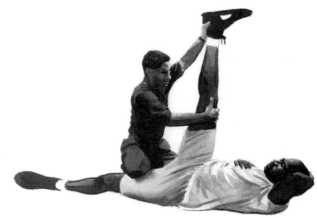

PIRIFORMIS STRETCH

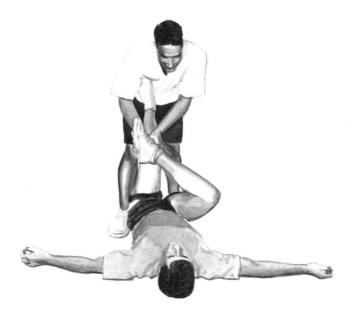

- Player, lying on back with both knees bent, takes right ankle and crosses it over on top of left knee (left foot is flat on floor).

- Partner places both hands on top of player's left knee and applies pressure to move player's left knee and right ankle toward chest.

Perform twice, holding each time, for 20 seconds

Repeat with left ankle across right knee

MUSCLES STRETCHED: piriformis, gluteals

I.T. BAND STRETCH (CROSSOVER)

- Player lies on his back with shoulder blades flat on floor.
- Partner slowly takes the player's right leg and crosses it over the other.
- Keep the opposite leg in place.
- The legs should be positioned at approximately 90° when the right leg is crossed over the left.

Perform twice, holding each time for 20 seconds
Repeat on the other leg

MUSCLES STRETCHED: tensor fasciae latae, gluteals, hamstring

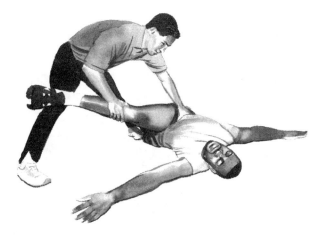

BUTTERFLY STRETCH

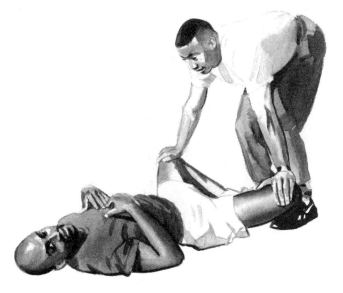

- Player lies on back with both knees bent, soles of feet together.
- Partner applies pressure on top of bent knees downward toward floor.

Perform twice, holding each time for 20 seconds

MUSCLES STRETCHED: thigh adductors

QUADRICEPS STRETCH (SINGLE LEG)

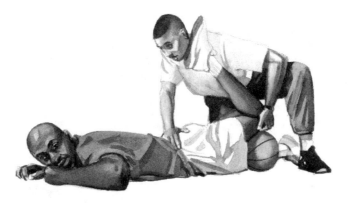

- Player lies on the floor, facedown with left leg bent and right leg straight.

- Partner places a basketball or a foot under player's bent knee. Slowly he lifts the player's left knee.

Perform twice, holding each time for 20 seconds
Repeat on the other leg

MUSCLES STRETCHED: quadriceps, iliopsoas, rectus femoris

CHEST (PECTORAL) STRETCH

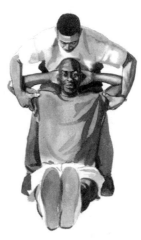

- Player, sitting, standing, or kneeling, places both hands behind his head.

- Partner, from behind, places both bent elbows into his hands and applies pressure by pulling elbows backward, behind the player's head.

Perform twice, holding each time for 20 seconds

MUSCLES STRETCHED: pectorals, anterior deltoids

SHOULDER/BICEP STRETCH

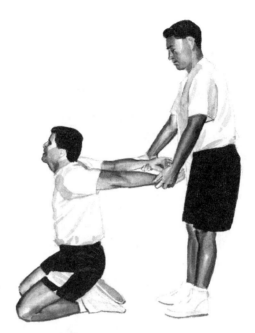

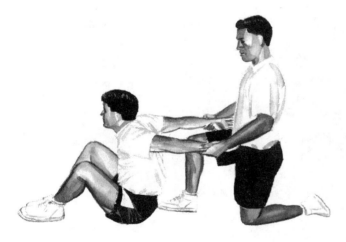

- Player is seated or kneeling.
- Partner takes both wrists into hands, palms facing up, and elevates the straight arms until the player feels the stretch.

Perform twice, holding each time for 20 seconds

MUSCLES STRETCHED: biceps, anterior deltoids, pectorals

GUIDELINES FOR PARTNER-STRETCHING

Either coach or athletes may perform the passive stretches.

- It is very important that proper technique be used throughout the movement.

- The stretcher should perform these movements slowly and with control.

- These stretches should not be painful, mild tension is the most the athlete should feel.

- The athlete should be stretched until he feels that it is a good stretch.

- More is not always better.

- The athlete being stretched and the stretcher (facilitator) should maintain constant verbal communication. This is to insure that the stretch is safe and adequate.

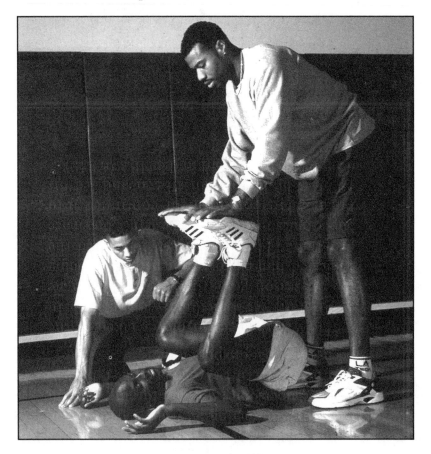

Loy Vaught of the **Los Angeles Clippers** is stretching his teammate **Gary Grant**. This lower back stretch is being closely watched by strength and conditioning coach **Carl Horne**.

PNF STRETCHING

PNF (proprioceptive neuromuscular facilitation) is an advanced form of passive stretching. There is now strong research evidence to support this form of stretching.

Once again, extreme care must be used by the coach or partner performing this style of stretching. We highly recommend that the coach or facilitator be skilled in stretching techniques and have enough knowledge of PNF to insure the safety of the athlete.

There are several preferred forms of PNF stretching techniques. The two most commonly used techniques by the strength and conditioning coaches of the NBA are *hold, contract, relax* and *contract, movement, relax.*

Here are examples of both techniques.

HOLD, CONTRACT, RELAX

An example of this is the PNF hamstring stretch. In performing *hold, contract, relax,* the athlete isometrically contracts his hamstring muscles while the coach pushes against the athlete's resistance. This isometric contraction is held for 5 to 10 seconds; followed by a 10-second relaxation period. After this *hold,* the athlete is stretched further. This cycle is repeated 3 times.

It is vital that the coach (or partner) talks to the athlete. For example, during the exercise, the coach may say to the athlete, "Hold against my resistance." Following this stretch, the coach gives the command, "Okay, now relax."

CONTRACT, MOVEMENT, RELAX

This technique is similar to the hold, contract, relax technique. Here the athlete attempts to push his leg toward the coach by contracting the hamstring muscles. The coach allows the leg to move in a predetermined range of motion before giving the "relax" command. During the relaxation phase, the coach moves the leg into a deeper stretched position and repeats. This cycle is also repeated 3 times.

MYTHS & MISCONCEPTIONS

Stretching is often misunderstood. As a result, it is performed improperly. Here are some common myths and misconceptions.

MYTH #1: STRETCHING IS EFFECTIVE ONLY WHEN IT HURTS.

Stretching should never "hurt." Stretching is a progressive activity that requires repeated practice sessions over a sustained period of time. Mild tension is the most an individual should experience. Actually, in order to gain significant improvement, your stretches should be held for longer lengths of time (15 to 20 seconds), and include multiple sets (2 to 3). After a short period (usually 2 weeks), your stretching will become much easier. Soon after that, it becomes an enjoyable and relaxing activity.

MYTH #2: STRETCHING IS NOT AS IMPORTANT AS WEIGHT-TRAINING OR RUNNING.

Stretching is just as important as any other aspect of a conditioning program. An athlete may be extremely strong, but only able to exhibit an average amount of power. This is most likely because he is inflexible. In most cases, the more an athlete can move his joints through a wider range of motion, the greater his power and effectiveness will be. This same athlete may also exhibit decreased running or leaping capabilities due to a shorter stride length.

MYTH #3: STRETCHING BEFORE PRACTICE WASTES VALUABLE PRACTICE TIME.

A sound stretching program should be included as part of practice. The first part of practice should be used to prepare athletes both physically and mentally for a vigorous practice session. This is also a valuable time for the team to come together and unify as a group.

MYTH #4: "WHY SHOULD I START STRETCHING? I'VE NEVER BEEN INJURED BEFORE."

As the old adage says, "Prevention is the best medicine." Some young athletes tend to be able to stay injury-free without stretching because their muscles, tendons and joints are already flexible. Once the physical maturation process begins in adolescence, muscle fibers lose some of their natural elasticity. This is the reason why it is especially important to stretch. Decreased flexibility leads to decreased performance and is also an indicator of aging.

You may be surprised to know that an athlete who stretches regularly can even improve his muscle elasticity with age. This is the reason why stretching programs should be initiated early on so that young athletes can learn proper techniques and develop good habits.

Remember: When you stretch, a muscle/tendon complex will only stretch to a certain limit; after that, when forces are great enough, the muscle will tear. Be sure this doesn't happen to you. Stretch safely. Don't try to accomplish too much in one session.

MYTH #5: IT'S BETTER TO BOUNCE WHILE I'M STRETCHING.

No, it's not better to bounce while stretching. During static stretching, muscles adapt after a period of time (15 to 20 seconds). Muscle, when held in a fixed stretched position, will adapt to that position and then relax. When repeated, the stretch will be further. If you bounce during a static stretch, the muscle can't learn the stretch and can't adapt.

MYTH #6: STRETCHING IS BAD FOR YOUR JOINTS.

Muscles, tendons, bones, cartilage, and ligaments control your joint stability and range of motion. Without good flexibility, your joint stability and range of motion will be diminished.

For example, tight hamstrings create increases in tension on the pelvic region and on the joints of the lower spine. This, in turn, causes a loss in joint ROM that can lead to increased pain, stiffness, and muscle spasms.

Stretching for the hamstrings and lower back must be a major concern and focus in conditioning for all athletes.

CONDITIONING

Each chapter of this book will help make you a better basketball player, but a proper conditioning base is the key. You need to look at conditioning as an opportunity to improve yourself as an athlete and a basketball player.

As a superior conditioned athlete, you can perform at higher intensities and sustain these efforts longer than someone that is not conditioned as well. Superior conditioning gives you an advantage and a better chance of winning.

In the summer of '92, **Gary Payton** of the **Seattle Supersonics** was at a turning point in his career. His first two years in the NBA had been somewhat disappointing.

He was the second player taken in the 1990 draft, yet something was missing. In the off-season going into his third year he dedicated himself to an intense conditioning program. That season (1993) he led the Supersonics to the NBA Western Conference Finals. His commitment continued into 1994 as he became an all-star and led his team to the best record in the NBA (63-19).

SCIENTIFIC INFORMATION

THE ENERGY SYSTEMS

There are three primary energy systems that your body uses during exercise. They are:

> ATP-CP System
> Glycogen Lactic Acid System
> Aerobic System

The ATP-CP system and the glycogen lactic acid systems are anaerobic. Basketball is a sport that requires repeated short high intensity efforts which utilize these anaerobic systems.

Each energy system is based on time of exercise. Listed below are the energy systems and the time utilized for each system. Note that one system does not shut off and another take over, but they work together during different time periods.

PRIMARY ENERGY SYSTEMS

```
                                          ATP-CP
                                   Glycogen Lactic Acid
ATP-CP<---------->Glycogen Lactic Acid<------------->Aerobic<----------------->Aerobic
```

Time:	10 seconds	1 minute	2 minutes	4 minutes	9 minutes	30 minutes	2 hours+
Distance:	100 yards	440 yards	880 yards	1 mile	2 miles	6 miles	marathon

This graph shows the three primary energy systems, and their exercise times and running distances. The connecting arrows between the three primary systems represent transition phases from one system to another. Only each extreme end of the graph is 100% anaerobic or aerobic metabolism for energy.

RECOVERY

Being able to recover quickly is critical for basketball players. Every player gets tired during intense practices and games, but well-conditioned athletes recover quicker and are able to continue high intensity effort throughout the practices and games.

SHORT-TERM RECOVERY

For well-conditioned athletes, the ATP-CP energy system is half recovered in about 20 to 30 seconds. (The rest during a free throw.) It is fully recovered in 2 to 5 minutes (the rest time during time outs, end of quarters, and when you are taken out of the game for a few minutes).

The glycogen lactic acid system is half recovered in about 20 to 30 minutes and is fully recovered in one hour or more. You will understand this when you start the conditioning program.

LONG-TERM RECOVERY

Long-term recovery can be from two days to several days depending on the extent of nutrient depletion, enzyme depletion, and tissue breakdown. Recovery, repair, and replenishment are aided by a good diet, proper rest and a quality training program.

Carbohydrates are the primary energy source used in the ATP-CP and glycogen lactic acid systems. For a more detailed discussion see the Nutrition chapter.

OFF-SEASON

The off-season is the time to prepare yourself physically for the demands of a long, intense season. The sport specific conditioning program should begin 12 weeks before the first day of basketball practice. It starts with 400 meter (440 yards) strides on a track and ends with sprints on the court. This program is two days per week and coincides with two days per week of plyometrics and agilities, which also will improve your conditioning level.

If you are involved in summer basketball leagues or other sports you will need to cut back a little in your conditioning, plyometrics, and agility programs or you will be overtraining. Signs of overtraining are feeling weaker in the weight room, not running as well on the track, or feeling run down or fatigued. You can cut back your conditioning program two ways:

1. Do just one day of conditioning and one day of plyometrics and agilities each week; or

2. Do all the days, but a little less each day.

ABOUT THE PROGRAM

The conditioning program starts with six weeks of strides. Starting with 400's (or 440's) working down to 100's (or 110's). Strides are good effort runs with smooth form. It is not a sprint and not $1/2$ speed, but about $3/4$ effort (see graph on on next page). Sprints start during week seven and are "all out efforts." The distances for sprints are 60 yards and less. Court work starts week eight and are also "all out efforts." The court work drills are explained on pages 54-56.

Each day's conditioning program is mapped out for you. The distances, number of repetitions, and the rest intervals are all set for you. Proper rest intervals are critical in developing your recovery system. It is suggested for best results, you should follow this plan.

For example, day 2 of week 2, after warming up and stretching out, you stride a 400—rest 3 minutes. Stride another 400—rest 3 minutes. This is repeated four times. After your last 400 you rest for 3 minutes and then start 200's. 200's have $11/2$ minutes rest between them. Repeat 4 of them and then cool down and stretch. Record your best 400 time and your best 200 time to monitor your progress.

PERCENTAGE ESTIMATION OF RUNNING SPEED

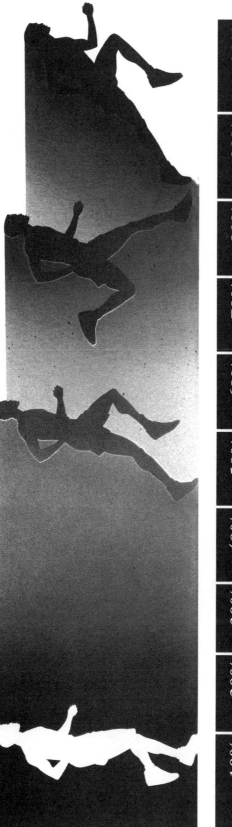

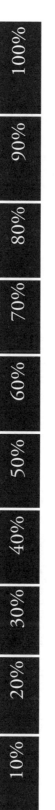

10%	20%	30%	40%	50%	60%	70%	80%	90%	100%

Jogging   Half Speed Stride   Three Quarter Speed Stride   Sprinting

OFF-SEASON
12-WEEK BASKETBALL-SPECIFIC
CONDITIONING PROGRAM

Week		Day	Drill	Distance	Rest Interval		Best Time
Week	1	Day 1	Stride	4 x 400	3	minutes	_____
		Day 2	Stride	4 x 400	3	minutes	_____
Week	2	Day 1	Stride	6 x 400	3	minutes	_____
		Day 2	Stride	4 x 400	3	minutes	_____
			Stride	4 x 200	$1^{1/2}$	minutes	_____
Week	3	Day 1	Stride	4 x 400	3	minutes	_____
			Stride	4 x 200	$1^{1/2}$	minutes	_____
		Day 2	Stride	4 x 400	3	minutes	_____
			Stride	6 x 200	$1^{1/2}$	minutes	_____
Week	4	Day 1	Stride	12 x 200	$1^{1/2}$	minutes	_____
		Day 2	Stride	12 x 200	$1^{1/2}$	minutes	_____
Week	5	Day 1	Stride	8 x 200	$1^{1/2}$	minutes	_____
			Stride	8 x 100	45	seconds	_____
		Day 2	Stride	8 x 200	$1^{1/2}$	minutes	_____
			Stride	8 x 100	45	seconds	_____
Week	6	Day 1	Stride	8 x 200	1	minute	_____
			Stride	8 x 100	30	seconds	_____
		Day 2	Stride	8 x 200	1	minute	_____
			Stride	8 x 100	30	seconds	_____

Week		Day	Drill	Distance	Rest Interval	Best Time
Week	7	Day 1	Stride	2 x 100	30 seconds	_____
			Stride	2 x 80	30 seconds	_____
			Sprint*	12 x 60	30 seconds	_____
		Day 2	Stride	2 x 100	30 seconds	_____
			Stride	2 x 80	30 seconds	_____
			Sprint	12 x 40	30 seconds	_____
Week	8	Day 1	Stride	2 x 100	30 seconds	_____
			Stride	2 x 80	30 seconds	_____
			Sprint	12 x 60	30 seconds	_____
		Day 2	COURT WORK			
			$5^{1/2}$'s x 2-3 times		$1^{1/2}$ minutes	_____
			Halfcourt, full court x 2-3 times		$1^{1/2}$ minutes	_____
			60-second side-line drill x 1**		(Do last)	_____
Week	9	Day 1	Stride	2 x 100	30 seconds	_____
			Stride	2 x 80	30 seconds	_____
			Sprint	12 x 40	25 seconds	_____
		Day 2	COURT WORK			
			$5^{1/2}$'s x 2-3		$1^{1/2}$ minutes	_____
			Halfcourt, full court x 2-3		$1^{1/2}$ minutes	_____
			60-second side-line drill x 2 times		3 minutes	_____
			Do in a circuit			

* Do not time yourself when sprinting, have a coach or friend time you.

** For 60-second side line drill record repetitions, not time.

Week			Day	Drill	Distance	Rest Interval	Best Time
Week	10		Day 1	Stride	2 x 100	30 seconds	_____
				Stride	2 x 80	30 seconds	_____
				Sprint	2 x 60	25 seconds	_____
				Sprint	2 x 40	25 seconds	_____
				Sprint	2 x 20	25 seconds	_____
				Sprint	4 x 10	25 seconds	_____
				Sprint	2 x 20	25 seconds	_____
				Sprint	2 x 40	25 seconds	_____
				Sprint	2 x 60	25 seconds	_____
			Day 2	COURT WORK			
				$5^{1/2}$'s x 2-4 times		$1^{1/2}$ minutes	_____
				Halfcourt, full court x 2-4 times		$1^{1/2}$ minutes	_____
				60-second side-line drill x 2 times		3 minutes	_____
Week	11		Day 1	$5^{1/2}$'s x 1		1 minute	_____
				Halfcourt, full court x 1		1 minute	_____
				Suicides x 2-3 times		1 minute	_____
				Reverse suicides x 2-3 times		1 minute	_____
				60-second side-line drill x 2 times		2 minutes	_____
			Day 2	$5^{1/2}$'s x 2 times		1 minute	_____
				Halfcourt, full court x 2 times		1 minute	_____
				Suicides x 2-4 times		1 minute	_____
				Reverse suicides x 2-4 times		1 minute	_____
				60-second side-line drill x 2 times		2 minutes	_____

Week		Day	Drill	Distance	Rest Interval	Best Time
Week	12	Day 1	5¹/₂'s x 2 times		1 minute	_____
			Halfcourt, full court x 2 times		1 minute	_____
			Suicides x 2-4 times		1 minute	_____
			Reverse suicides x 2-4 times		1 minute	_____
			60-second sideline drill x 2 times		2 minutes	_____
		Day 2	5¹/₂'s x 2 times		1 minute	_____
			Halfcourt, full court x 2 times		1 minute	_____
			Suicides x 2-4 times		1 minute	_____
			Reverse suicides x 2-4 times		1 minute	_____
			60-second sideline drill x 2 times		2 minutes	_____

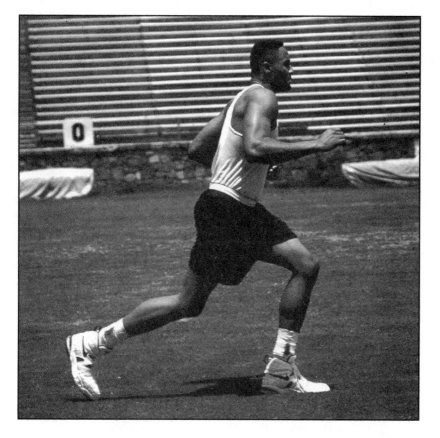

Alonzo Mourning of the **Charlotte Hornets** doing his conditioning work on a football field.

COURT WORK DRILLS

5¹/₂'S

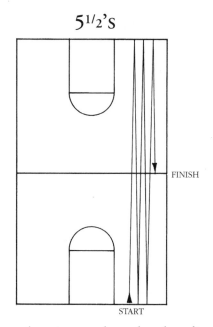

Start at one baseline and sprint to the other baseline. Repeat this five times and finish at halfcourt. Stay in a straight line.

HALFCOURT, FULL COURT

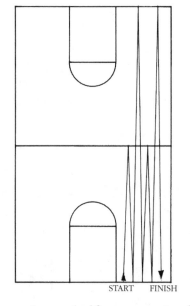

Start at one baseline, sprint to halfcourt, sprint back to the baseline. Then sprint to the other baseline, sprint back, and sprint to halfcourt. Sprint back again, sprint to the other baseline, and sprint back. Stay in a straight line.

60-SECOND SIDELINE DRILL

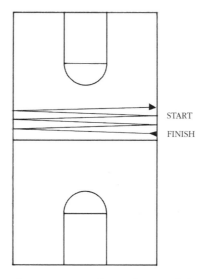

Start at one sideline and sprint to the other sideline and back. Repeat as many times as possible in 60 seconds. Over and back is 2 repetitions. Try to achieve 17 or more repetitions. Stay in a straight line.

SUICIDES

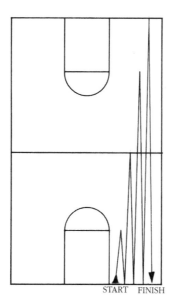

Start at the baseline, sprint to the free-throw line, and sprint back to the baseline. Then sprint to halfcourt, sprint back to the baseline, sprint to the other free-throw line and back. Finally sprint to the other baseline and back. Stay in a straight line.

REVERSE SUICIDES

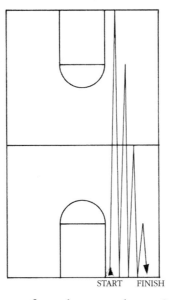

START   FINISH

These are like suicides, but go from long to short. Start at the baseline and sprint to the other baseline and back. Then sprint to the far free-throw line and back. Sprint to halfcourt and back. Then sprint to the closer free-throw line and back to the baseline.

RUNNING STAIRS

For variety in your court work conditioning program you may run stairs as an option if they are available. Repetitions will depend on the total number of stairs. Suggested repetitions: 10 to 20.

CONDITIONING DURING OTHER SEASONS

PRE-SEASON

Our definition of pre-season is the time between the first practice in the fall until the first game. This is the time your coach fine-tunes your off-season conditioning into quality basketball conditioning. If you followed the off-season program, you'll go into pre-season in very good shape. That way you can concentrate on basketball and not struggle with your conditioning.

IN-SEASON

During basketball season, a conditioning program consists of quality practices and intense games. If your practice consists of intense all-out drills, running the court hard, and good-quality defensive work, you don't need extra conditioning.

If not, you can do extra on-court conditioning drills from the off-season conditioning program. This also holds true for games if you're not getting much playing time.

POST-SEASON

Most basketball teams including most middle schools, high schools and colleges end their basketball season in March. The time immediately after a season is called the post-season. The post-season is the "active rest" time of the year. Initially, you will recover physically from a long basketball season. Some young athletes may go right into a spring sport such as baseball, tennis, or track. Others may be in true active rest.

During post-season you should stay fit by playing other sports or by working out in the beginning phase of the weight-training program. If you are not getting much running from other sports or pick up games from basketball you need to do some general fitness activities such as biking, jogging, swimming, or hiking. Conditioning machines such as stair climbers, rowers, or bikes would also be an option. You need to spend 20 to 40 minutes on these exercise conditioning machines. Jogging should be about 2 miles. This should be done 2 to 3 times per week.

AGILITY

For an aspiring young athlete, the best way to reach new levels of basketball performance is to develop yourself into a well-rounded athlete. This is true whether you are trying to make your high school squad, earn a college scholarship, or aspire to the highest level of basketball—the NBA.

All levels of basketball competition, from grade school up to the pros, demand the same sort of movements from every player. They must sprint, change direction, get "off the mark," turn and go, explode vertically once-twice-three times, speed up at various angles, and move from side to side with sudden bursts of speed in opposite directions. The combinations of these movements are endless because the game is so unpredictable.

A player's ability to *read and react* in any given offensive or defensive situation is the essence of basketball intelligence. Your ability to apply a specific basketball skill in any game is determined by your being able to move your body quickly and efficiently.

Agility refers to being able to change your body direction quickly, explosively, efficiently, and in balance (under control). Just as shooting foul shots is a highly technical skill requiring hours of disciplined practice, so is agility. Players who can't make changes quickly will no doubt struggle at both ends of the floor, especially as the opposing players improve their agility. This brings us to an unwritten rule in basketball:

FOR EVERY LEVEL YOU GO UP IN COMPETITION,
YOUR WEAKNESSES WILL BE MAGNIFIED ANOTHER DEGREE.

There is no question that agility training must be an integral part of building a well-rounded athlete. In order to get the job done, you must practice your basketball abilities both on and off the court.

SPEED, POWER, BALANCE

For better understanding of agility conditioning, it is necessary to recognize that basketball demands that movements be executed in a dynamic, explosive, and repetitive way. Therefore agility involves:

SPEED — The ability to move your body from one point to another running at 90 to 100 percent of your capacity.

POWER — The ability to exert force in the shortest possible time (see Plyometrics chapter for Power Formula)

BALANCE — The ability to regulate shifts in your body's center of gravity while maintaining control

These components must be practiced regularly with a great deal of dedication and commitment if you are seriously interested in developing yourself as a basketball player. No one characteristic is more important than the other. Agility involves the synergy of speed, power, and balance.

Synergy means that the whole effect is greater than the sum of its parts. For example, an athlete may be performing an agility skill by exhibiting both speed and power; but if he is "out of control" (not in balance), he is not performing that particular agility skill to the best of his potential.

By practicing the drills in the Speed and Plyometrics sections in this book, you will greatly increase your own agility. Be sure to work on the Speed exercises that focus on starting ability, acceleration, stride frequency, and stride length. In the Plyometrics section, make sure you emphasize working on lateral movements, changes of direction, and vertical jumps. These exercises will begin to create highly efficient and more agile movements for you.

Essential to basketball is leg strength. Your lower extremities must be conditioned thoroughly. The importance of a strong trunk (upper-body) area (including the lower back and abdominal muscles) must be emphasized strongly. This area serves as a stabilizer to your lower extremities, and must be conditioned thoroughly. As a result, your leg and hip area will move more independently. And you'll be able to move much more quickly and explosively.

LATERAL AGILITY

Basketball players must be able to move laterally quickly and smoothly. This is due to the fact that lateral moves (step/drag or slide) initiate so many changes in direction. To improve laterally, you must train laterally. Just as a sprinter can improve only by practicing movements at high rates of speed, a basketball player must focus on practicing his lateral agility.

Athletes must condition all body parts with equal attention and care. The weight-training exercises make your muscles stronger and plyometric exercises make your muscles more powerful. Agility training will make you move quicker and more efficiently.

Lack of proper conditioning places an athlete under risk of injury. Be sure that, in all your drills, you focus on quality. This is true whether you happen to be moving straight ahead, backward, sideways, or in an upward direction.

LEVELS AND PLANES OF PLAY

The game of basketball requires players to display a variety of complex movements. Basketball requires you to use your legs, arms, and hands, and it calls for a combination of speed and endurance, jumping and agility beyond most other sports. Players must move through a number of horizontal and vertical planes. Each of these moves involves many factors. For example, lateral movement requires three things:

- that your hips move abduct and adduct, and flex and extend;
- that you flex and extend your knee joints; and
- that your ankle dorsi-flex, plantar-flex, evert and invert.

In basketball a player must often turn halfway around before breaking into a full sprint. Requiring the player to quickly turn his whole body, agility is necessary for every good basketball player.

TEACHING TECHNIQUES

You will make the best progress by first performing the drills at a slow speed. This way you can master your technical form. From there, you can move to higher rates of speed. There's an important rule to follow here: Never sacrifice technique for speed.

Essentially what we need to do is "teach the feet" what to do. Using the ground is required in order to produce force; you must plant your feet fully on the ground—not just push off with your toes. This is true whether you start from a static ready position or change direction at full speed. You must have total foot contact with the ground's surface in order to produce the most power.

Starting high on your toes is never as powerful. The less contact your foot has with the surface, the less power you'll create. Don't sit back on your heels either. Let your feet be in full contact with the ground. Your body weight should lean slightly forward onto the ball of the foot. This action permits you to "push off" powerfully with the balls of your feet.

Basketball requires players to make hundreds of unpredictable foot patterns during every game. Therefore, attaining the utmost foot power will allow you to utilize a full range of basketball skills.

When moving straight ahead, backward, or laterally, you must try to push the ground "away" from yourself. Spend as little time in the air as possible. This produces as few vertical components in your stride as possible. If you want to learn a lot about this technique, watch another player's head. If it stays level, his form is fine; if you notice any "bobbing" action, it isn't.

Keep your knees flexed and situated over your toes, but never extend them fully. Your hips will move and, most importantly, should not settle too close to the ground when you come to a full stop or change direction. Let your trunk remain "tall" and sit just over your hips.

Do this without any excess leaning forward/backward or rocking. This ensures that your body's center of gravity will remain in the most efficient position possible while producing the most efficient movement possible.

Each sport is unique in regard to movement patterns. Fortunately, many of these can be "rehearsed" before competition. For instance, a tennis player can rehearse moving to the forehand side, hitting the ball, and then recovering back to center. The shortstop can rehearse going into the deep hole in either direction. The volleyball player can rehearse advancing to the net, and then backing off.

Many of these movements have their own natural "rhythm" and can be rehearsed hundreds of times prior to competition. Try practicing your movements in slow motion. This way you give yourself enough time to work on improving your technique, balance, coordination, and concentration.

You will almost immediately integrate the synergistic effects of this practice into your full skills repertoire. For an agility program, you must devise drills that will:

- be of short duration (anaerobic);

- produce at least 2 or 3 directional changes;

- focus on lateral movement;

- mix lateral with straight-ahead and backpedaling movements, thus producing quick rotations;

- produce a "counter-move": a 1 to 2 foot slide or hop in one direction; follow this by working (sprint/slide) in the opposite direction;

- demand ankle agility.

TRAINING SCHEDULE

You will probably produce your greatest results in agility conditioning during the off- and pre-season periods. During these times you can work at your highest intensity and still allow for sufficient recovery time.

Of course every athlete hopes to create a strong "carryover" effect into the regular season. Nevertheless, you should be able to at least maintain your off-season progress throughout the regular season.

If you receive a lot of game and practice time, you'll find it relatively easy to maintain your high level of conditioning. If you receive limited playing time, you must put in extra work before and/or after practice in order to maintain your progress.

AGILITY WORKOUT: INDIVIDUAL AND TEAM

COMPLETE THE SQUARE

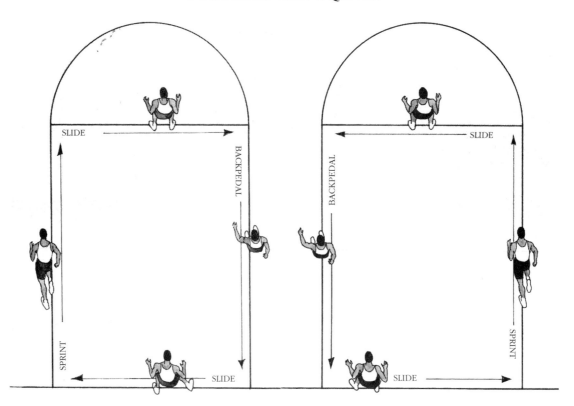

- Player starts in a ready position at the corner of the left side of the free-throw line.

- 4 consecutive trips are made around the lane: 2 clockwise (trips 1 & 3) and 2 counterclockwise trips (trips 2 & 4).

- On "Go," player sprints forward down the lane. Upon reaching the edge of the baseline and lane, he then slides to the right until he reaches the opposite lane line. He backpedals up the lane to the right edge of the free-throw line and then slides left back to the starting position.

- Once he reaches the starting point, he reverses direction and repeats drill in opposite way.

- After completing 1 clockwise trip and 1 counterclockwise trip, you repeat the movement.

- 4 total trips around lane count as one drill.

COMPLETE THE SQUARE, WITH JUMP ROPE

- Player starts in ready jump-rope position at the corner of the left side of the free-throw line.

- 2 consecutive trips are made around the lane; 1 clockwise (trip 1) and 1 counterclockwise (trip 2).

- *Forward* Player works down the lane, moving forward in any number of foot patterns of choice with the jump rope.

    - Soft pitter pat run
    - Double leg soft hop
    - Single leg soft hop
    - Single leg soft hop at 45° angles

- *Side* Upon reaching the edge of the baseline and lane, player works to the right again, using any of the following foot patterns:

    - Double leg soft hop to the right
    - Single leg (right or left) soft hop
    - High knees working to the right

- *Back* Upon reaching the opposite edge of the lane, player works backward up the lane, using any of the following patterns:

    - Soft backpedal
    - Double leg soft hop backward
    - High knees backward

- *Side* At the right edge of the foul line, player works any of the side movements already listed above, moving back to start. Once he reaches the start, he reverses direction (counterclockwise) and works the same pattern of his choice. Your goal for the 2 trips is to complete both trips without stopping.

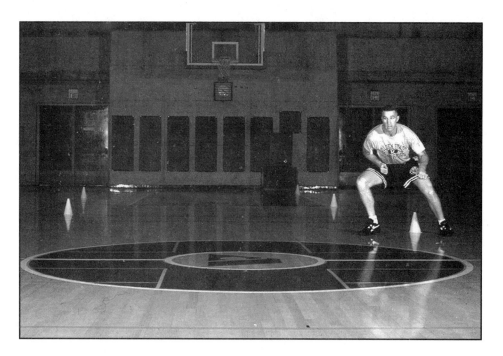

Chris Mullin of the **Golden State Warriors** is doing
an angled agility drill with cones.

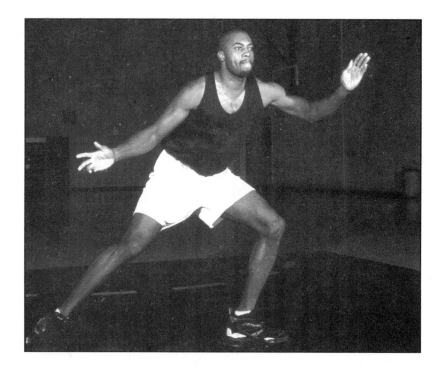

Glen Rice of the **Miami Heat** is working
on improving his agility.

STAR RUNS IN THE LANE

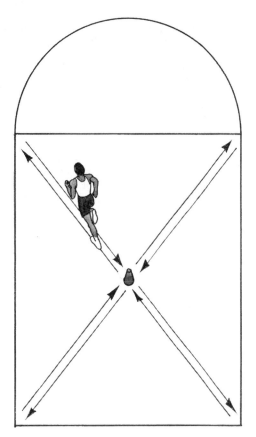

- Player places a marker (tape or cone) in the center of the foul lane.

- Player starts in a ready position, then races to any corner of the lane. He races back to the center, then moves on to next corner of his choice until all four corners are completed.

- Do two repetitions each of the following five different foot patterns:

    – Sprint forward to corner, sprint back to center

    – Backpedal to corner, sprint forward to center

    – Slide laterally to corner, slide back to center

    – Slide to corner, sprint back to center

    – Sprint to corner, slide back to center

RICOCHET PICKUPS

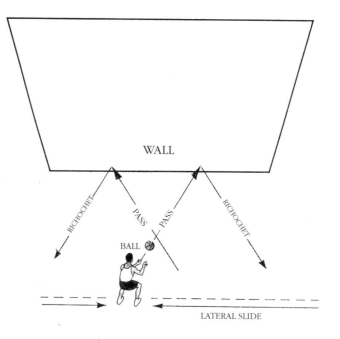

- Standing 3 to 5 yards from a wall, player with ball in both hands assumes a ready athletic position, feet spread slightly wider than normal. Ball is held low, close to floor.

- Player plays ball low off the wall at an angle and slides laterally to retrieve it, but never crosses his feet. Once ball is caught, he then plays ball off the wall to the other side and slides to retrieve it. He continues to work side to side.

- Ball must be played low (1 to $1^1/_2$ feet) off the wall so that it has a rolling effect as it comes back to player.

- Don't chest pass off the wall, but try to throw it underhand, with 2 hands always catching and passing.

Duration: 10 to 15 seconds
Changes of direction during drill: 4 to 6
Intensity: Low-maximum (depending on phase)
Recovery time: 30 to 60 seconds (depending on intensity)
Number of repetitions: 6 to 12 (depending on phase)

LATERAL SLIDE WITH RESPONSE

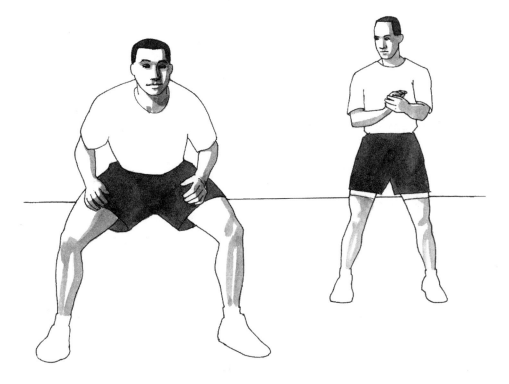

- Standing at the free throw line, player assumes a ready athletic position with coach standing behind player. (Player faces away from coach.)

- On "Go," player slides right laterally toward the sideline without crossing his feet.

- Upon hearing the coach clap, player changes direction quickly toward the other sideline and keeps changing direction whenever he hears a clap.

- Coach tries to sound a clap in an unpredictable manner to keep athlete ready to change direction quickly and at any time.

- Drill can be done with one player or with full team. If done with full team, break team in half. One half works while the other rests.

Duration: 8 to 10 seconds
Changes of direction during drill: 4 to 6
Intensity: Low-maximum (depending on phase)
Recovery time: 30 to 60 seconds (depending on intensity)

Number of repetitions: 6 to 12 (depending on phase)

THE WHEEL

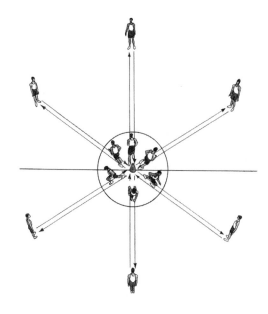

- Pair up a larger and smaller player (6 pairs).

- If you have fewer players, you can use cones.

- Set each pair in a circle 7 to 10 yards equidistant from the center jump circle.

- Have smaller players walk to center with larger players staying in place serving as outside markers.

- On "Go" all smaller players will then sprint to their partners first, touch hand of partner, then sprint back to center. After completion of the first run they will continue on in a clockwise fashion touching all six outside markers, always returning to the center after each outside marker is touched. All smaller players run at same time and the drill is complete when all of them finish in center circle.

- Smaller players now replace the larger players as markers on outside and larger players perform drill.

VARIATIONS OF THE WHEEL

1. Face into center circle and backpedal to and around partner then sprint back to center.

2. Defensive slides around marker, then sprint back to center.

GASSER ROTATIONS

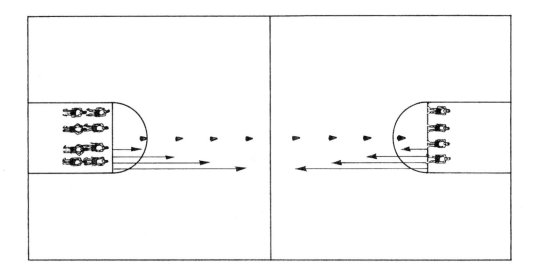

- Break team into three groups of equal speed ability.

- Line one group along one free throw line.

- Line the other two groups at the opposite foul line with one group behind the other group.

- Place 3 or 4 cones in a straight line about 2 to $2^{1}/2$ yards from the foul line then string out cones.

- Foul lines serve as starting positions.

- Drill begins with the first of two groups at one end sprinting to first cone, racing back to the foul line then sprinting to second cone and back to foul line until all the cones at one end have been used. After completion of cone drill, this group will sprint to the resting group at the opposite foul line. Once the working group passes the foul line, the next group will perform the same drill at the other end. Upon completion they will then sprint to the final group who perform the same drill to complete the rotation.

- Groups will do 6 to 10 rotations. This gives a 1:2 work/rest ratio during the drill.

VARIATIONS OF FOOT SKILLS FOR GASSER ROTATIONS DRILL

1.   Sprint to cone, turn and sprint back to foul line.

2.   Sprint to cone, backpedal to foul line.

3.   Sprint to cone, defensive 45° slides to foul line.

4.   Lateral slide to cone, lateral slide back to foul line.

5.   Lateral slide to cone, sprint back to foul line.

6.   Sprint to cone, lateral slide to foul line.

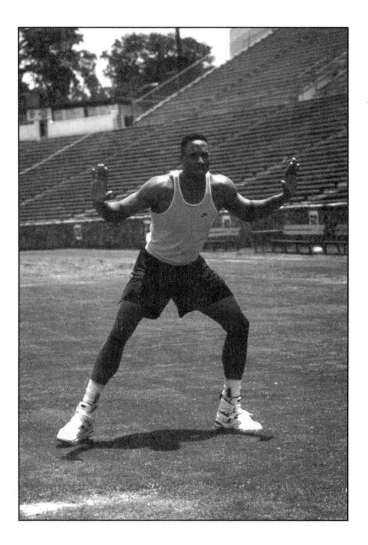

Alonzo Mourning of the **Charlotte Hornets**
is working on his lateral movement.

QUESTIONS & ANSWERS

1. When is the best time during the week for agility drills?

This depends on the particular phase of your training schedule. The Off-Season Total Program (see Putting It All Together), suggests agility drills be performed on Monday and Thursday.

2. How long should each drill take?

Most agility exercise should take no longer than 10 seconds. They are predominantly anaerobic and should be performed at maximum speed and intensity for the best development. If fatigue sets in, stop the drill until you have adequately recovered for the next bout.

3. Is there a time of year when I don't have to devote as much time to agility work?

Yes, during the in-season with games and practices you still incorporate agility skills because you are now practicing the specific skills you prepared for in the off-season. Plus the intensity levels are always at their highest during games and practices.

4. How do I know if I'm doing the drills technically correct?

The watchful eye of a coach is best; he or she can spot any flaws. Also, the use of a video is an excellent tool. Have someone videotape your practice and then review it with your coach.

5. Can I do agility work without doing weight-training and plyometrics?

Weight-training and plyometrics are two areas that surely enhance your movements skills as well as prevent injury. They both strengthen and condition the vital areas (hips, legs, ankles) that become stressed during intense agility work and accelerate your improvement in movement.

PLYOMETRICS

You may have heard of plyometrics but you may not know what it is. Plyometrics involves exercises that put your muscles on a rapid pre-stretch before an explosive contraction. These explosive movements include jumping, bounding, power skips, and hops.

Plyometric training is actually very demanding on your body and can have a dramatic impact on your athletic performance.

THE POWER FORMULA

The ability to generate power is critical to successful athletic performance.

What is power? Power is the relationship between strength (force) and speed, or, more precisely:

$$\text{POWER} = \text{FORCE} \ \text{x} \ \frac{\text{DISTANCE}}{\text{TIME}}$$

Strength is a major component of the power formula. Strength is the ability of a muscle to exert force. Unfortunately, too often an athlete is thought to be strong only if he can lift a lot of poundage in the weight room. This is referred to as "absolute strength" and is of little value if it's not readily transferable to the sporting arena.

The truly powerful athlete is one who is able to incorporate maximum force in the shortest time possible. Power, therefore, is the ability to exert force in an explosive manner. This force may involve one of two things: either the timely contraction of the muscles that extend the ankles, knees, hips, and shoulders just before a vertical jump; or the force generated by a coordinated contraction of the chest, shoulders, and triceps during a basketball chest pass.

VARIETY OF MOVEMENTS

Forward, backward, lateral, and vertical sprints, shuffles, slides, skips and hops are many of the movements you may experience in a typical basketball game. The position of every basketball player on the floor changes from moment to moment. As a result, you must continually adjust to fit each circumstance.

Since basketball requires this variety of movement patterns, your conditioning program must focus on developing movement variety. The information in this book will help develop such skills; your coach can also help.

A coach can design plyometric drills based on your individual needs. You may employ specific movement drills that closely resemble movement patterns unique to that athlete's particular sport and position. Or you may choose to incorporate basic movement patterns found in other sports. These include lateral, forward, backward, vertical, and rotational movements, and combinations thereof. For example, an athlete who has difficulty moving left and right may need drills that place greater emphasis on explosive lateral movements.

Coaches and athletes alike should be reassured that the variety of plyometric drills available is unlimited; therefore, you are encouraged to create your own drills to accommodate all situations. This variety will also help you to prevent athletic burn out by changing the drill patterns and training routine regularly.

Use common sense; approach any new activity with caution. Try out your new drills and exercises carefully before you or anyone else goes at it full steam ahead.

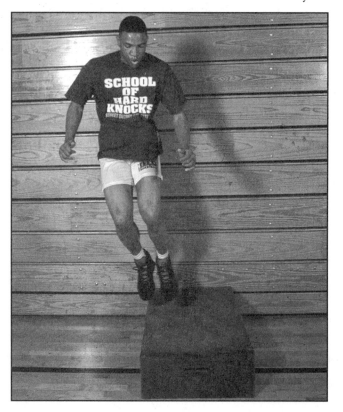

Doc Rivers of the **New York Knicks** is working on lateral box jumps.

"DOC" RIVERS ON PLYOMETRICS

When **"Doc" Rivers** was traded to the **New York Knicks** for the '92-'93 season, the media and the fans questioned the wisdom of the move. Most thought he was on the last leg of his NBA career. Doc was considered half a step too slow because of his age. His post-season ('92 -'93) conditioning test scores were fair, but not outstanding. For example:

- his sit and reach flexibility was measured at +5.5 inches;
- his 20-yard agility sprint was 4.67 seconds;
- his standing vertical jump was 28 inches; and
- his vertical jump with an approach step was 32 inches.

After three months of off-season training with the Knicks, Doc improved his performance field test scores considerably. How? By his commitment to his plyometric exercises.

Doc improved:

- his flexibility improved an inch;
- his agility sprint time dropped from 4.67 to 4.35 seconds;
- his standing vertical jump improved 2 inches;
- his vertical jump with an approach step soared to 36 inches, a 4-inch improvement.

SAFETY CONSIDERATIONS

Before you start, a word of caution. Plyometric training is not for everyone! The exercises and degree of difficulty you choose must be right for your own body. They cannot be expected to compare with the exercises and degree of difficulty chosen by older, more experienced athletes. Consult your physician and coach before beginning plyometric training.

The following will tell you what you need to know before you begin.

Young athlete	Young athletes—even a first-year high school student, for example—should be strictly supervised. There's always a chance that an injury could occur. Young athletes are more likely to injure a joint or damage a growth plate in the bones. Therefore, they should be given only those exercises that are listed as "low intensity" and "low impact."
Intensity	You should approach a plyometric workout with caution. Just because an exercise looks easy, doesn't mean it *is* easy. Plyometric exercises should go from the less difficult to the more advanced drills. That way your body will adapt in the most efficient manner.
Medical history	If you have a history of injuries, or are currently recovering from an injury, you should stay away from plyometrics. Only after obtaining a doctor or trainer's release should an injured athlete resume plyometric conditioning.
Surface	The surface for plyometrics should be semi-resilient—bouncy, but not too bouncy. Good basketball courts, tumbling mats, a rubberized track, and dry, well-groomed grass usually provide excellent surfaces.
Footwear	Shoes should be worn at all times. Basketball shoes are preferable. They provide good lateral stability, heel cushion, arch support, and non-slip soles.

Equipment

Boxes should be strong and sturdy. There should be no protruding objects such as handles on the top or sides of the boxes. Boxes should vary in height from 3 inches to 3 feet. Cover the box with a smooth, not a shaggy, carpet. The carpet gives the box some padding, but it doesn't slow down your movement. It should be glued to the box and shouldn't cause too much friction on the bottom of your shoe.

Don't cover the box with rubber matting. It may feel soft under your foot, but your rubber sole will tend to stick to the rubber matting at the moment you try to jump. Some drills require a slight twisting action. If you try to twist or pivot while in contact with a rubber-topped box, a joint injury could occur.

Barriers

Barriers should never be the source of an injury to the athlete. Use foam barriers or a couple of rolled-up towels with a piece of tape wrapped around them works well.

Medicine balls

They are extremely useful when trying upper- (and lower-) body plyometrics. Inflatable rubber medicine balls work the best because they rebound when they hit the floor or the wall. Medicine balls should weigh from 2 to 15 pounds.

Spotting

As the drills become harder it is important that at least one person stands ready to spot potential problems before an injury happens. Other athletes turn out to be the best spotters since they know exactly what the early warning signs of exhaustion look like. Spotting should be taught as an integral part of their plyometric training.

SIX GUIDELINES FOR ATHLETES

1. STRENGTH BASE

It's very important that you understand your level of strength before you begin a plyometric program. Sufficient strength is critical since it will permit you to use the correct drill technique, and thereby reduce the risk of injury. Coaches can assess strength improvements by continual observation and selected standards of measurement. These can indicate whether or not you are ready to advance to the next level of drill difficulty.

Plyometrics is best employed when combined with weight training. These drills are by no means a replacement for a strength program. Remember, power is the relationship between strength and speed. Therefore, the stronger the athlete, the greater the potential for increased power development. As your strength levels improve, you may progress to higher intensity drills.

2. WARM-UP, STRETCHING, AND COOL-DOWN

A comprehensive warm-up, stretching, and cool-down program is necessary before and after a training session. Jogging, easy strides, calisthenics, and low-key skipping are examples of warm-up activities.

The active warm-up is followed by a total body stretching routine. After the training session has been completed, you should again perform some low-intensity active cool-down activities, and finish off the session by stretching again. Please refer to the Warming Up, Stretching, Cooling Down chapter.

3. PROGRESSION

Plyometrics, like other high-intensity activities, are typically performed immediately following the warm-up routine and before other exercise methods which may be scheduled for that particular training session. Since the training focus of plyometrics is neuromuscular, fatigue can have a negative impact, especially for the less-well-developed athlete. Therefore, plyometrics should be performed at highest intensity when you are "fresh." This will decrease the chance of injury.

Discontinue the drill as soon as you reach a point of moderate fatigue. Always maintain proper technique in order to achieve maximum gain and decrease the chance of injury. Of equal importance is adequate rest between sets and sessions. This allows your body time to recover and ultimately adapt to the physical stress imposed.

4. INTENSITY

When performing plyometrics, you should be focused and attentive to the purpose of the drill and the technique required. Intensity levels are basically determined by the degree of impact within a particular drill. As a general rule, the following drills are categorized as high-intensity plyometrics exercises:

- Significant displacement of the body's center of gravity; this means covering a lot of horizontal ground per hop, skip, or bound

- Take-off and landing on a single leg

- Absorbing the body's impact from a drop height of greater than 12 inches

- Skills or exercises requiring advanced movement coordination

HIGH-INTENSITY DRILLS

- Single leg hops for distance

- Depth jumps from the tops of boxes

- Bounding

- High barrier jumps

LOW-INTENSITY DRILLS

- Low vertical and horizontal displacement

- Double leg jumps in place

- Relatively easy movement coordination

- Running in place

- Skipping rope

- Side to side jumps over a small barrier

It is important for the beginner to establish a solid technical understanding before advancing on to higher intensity drills. Drill intensity will vary depending upon your physical maturity level. For example, the degree of impact (and therefore the intensity level) would be significantly greater for a 200-pound athlete performing a simple depth jump off a 12-inch box, than the same drill performed by a 130-pound athlete. Care must be taken not to lump all athletes into one category. A progressive coach is sympathetic to each athlete's individual needs and adjusts the training sessions accordingly.

5. EXERCISE DIFFICULTY

Exercise difficulty is closely associated with intensity. Many drills and exercises outwardly appear to be easy and have a low intensity. It is in these precise exercises that you must take special care not to overindulge. Too often, you may not feel it until the next morning when you roll out of bed; and by then it's too late.

Plyometrics are extremely demanding on your body. As a result, you should carefully follow a program that gradually progresses from beginning to advanced exercises. Beginners should build a base by performing flat-surfaced, double-leg and low impact drills. Once you develop a strength base, more demanding exercises such as single-leg, tall barrier, and higher impact drills can be incorporated into your program.

6. REPETITIONS, SETS, AND SESSIONS

The number of repetitions and sets varies depending on the intensity of the drill. Generally, a low intensity exercise would require a higher number of repetitions. Likewise, an exercise with a higher degree of difficulty would result in lower repetitions. The number of drills to perform will also vary. You should not exceed six high-impact exercises during any one plyometric workout. The total volume of repetitions will be determined by the number of exercises you perform, the number of sets per drill, and the degree of difficulty. To allow for full recovery of your muscles, tendons, and ligaments (which become stressed during a plyometric workout), a two- or three-day rest period (48-hour minimum) between sessions provides optimal results.

BEGINNING PLYOMETRICS TRAINING

LENGTH
- 12 weeks
- 1 to 2 sessions per week
- 15 to 30 minutes per session

RECOVERY
- 48 to 72 hours minimum between sessions
- 2 to 4 minutes between sets

REPS/SETS
- 80 to 120 total repetitions per upper and/or lower body per session

INTENSITY
- Low

IN-SEASON PLYOMETRICS TRAINING

LENGTH
- Varies depending on the length of the season, competition schedule, practice intensity, and minutes played during a game
- 1 to 2 sessions per week
- 15 to 30 minutes per session

RECOVERY
- 48-hour minimum between sessions
- 1 to 3 minutes between sets

REPS/SETS
- Repetitions per upper and /or lower body per session

    Young athlete: 25 to 75 repetitions
    Mature athlete: 50 to 100 repetitions

INTENSITY
- Low to moderate

Note: In-season plyometrics training is to be done by athletes not getting much playing time. Be careful not to overtrain.

POST-SEASON PLYOMETRICS TRAINING

LENGTH
- 4 weeks after the end of the in-season
- Intensity, frequency, and duration of training sessions drop considerably
- Time should be spent in "active rest" type activities

OFF-SEASON PLYOMETRICS TRAINING

LENGTH
- Varies, depending upon competition schedule
- 2 to 3 sessions per week
- 30 to 45 minutes per session

RECOVERY
- 48 hours minimum between sessions
- 1 to 2 minutes between sets

REPS/SETS
- Total repetitions per upper and/or lower body per session

  Novice athlete: 100 to 150 repetitions
  Mature athlete: 150 to 200 repetitions

INTENSITY
- Moderate to high

QUESTIONS & ANSWERS

1. How can I improve my vertical jump?

Vertical and horizontal jumping are power activities. Power is a relationship between speed and strength. To improve your vertical jump, you should first strengthen the specific muscles involved in the movement. For example, the major muscles involved in vertical jumping include the calves, hamstrings, gluteals, quadriceps, and shoulders (strong abdominal and low back muscles are also important).

Possessing strength is only part of the total picture. Jumping improves jumping. To improve your vertical jump, practice vertical jumping. Combine the drills outlined in this chapter with a comprehensive strength training program and you'll see significant gains in your vertical jump ability.

2. I've seen athletes jumping off boxes 4 feet high. Will I see faster results if I do the same?

More is not always better. None of our professional players jump off boxes higher than 18 inches. Most use boxes ranging from 9 to 12 inches. We are more concerned with the speed of the jump rather than the height of the drop. This is true since the risk of injury far outweighs the potential for physical improvements. We frequently perform a considerable number of tests on the players (i.e., vertical jump, horizontal jump, agility sprint). And we continually see improvements in our test results and on the court.

THE PLYOMETRICS WORKOUT

Before starting your own routine, carefully pick the movement patterns you need. Concentrate on those drills that are right for you. Make sure you become good in performing the basic movements before tackling harder ones.

Now for the drills themselves. Here are a few that creative coaches and athletes have developed over the years. But there are literally hundreds of combinations of plyometric exercises. Once you catch on, we encourage you to create your own drills.

PLEASE NOTE: One repetition equals one full completion of the exercise. For example, if you perform a simple jump in place, each time your feet make contact with the floor, count one repetition. If an exercise requires multiple movements such as side-to-side barrier jumps, then count one complete "round trip" (i.e. over and back) as one repetition.

REMEMBER: Carelessness can lead to an injury—
so use good judgment.

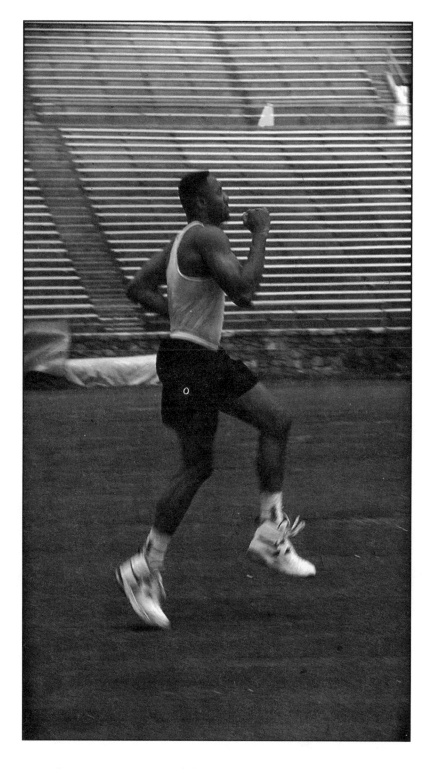

Alonzo Mourning of the **Charlotte Hornets** is doing
the plyometric exercise called bounding.

RIM JUMPS

As the name implies, you jump up and try to touch touch the rim. If you can't reach the rim, then perhaps try to get as high as the bottom of the backboard, the net, or any other suspended object. This drill is a series of rapid vertical jumps. You should concentrate on being quick off the ground. A good phrase to remember is "touch and go."

The speed of the jump is more important than the height; however, always encourage yourself to make maximum vertical effort.

- Assume an upright stance, eyes focused on the target.

- Start by quickly dropping to a quarter squat position—ankles, knees, hips, shoulders, and elbows are flexed.

- Immediately jump and reach to the target (with one hand).

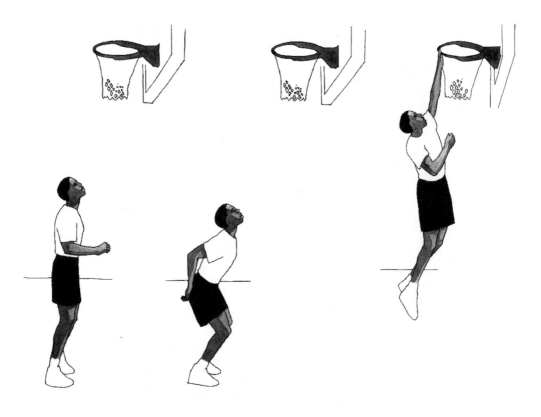

CONDITIONING TIP: After you attain your peak height and begin your descent, you should start thinking about the next jump before hitting the ground. In other words, elbows, shoulders, hips, and knees should be flexed and ready for the next jump.

KNEES TO ELBOWS

This drill is like the rim jump. It requires you to jump to maximum height, your hips and knees flexed during the flight phase, while maintaining quickness off the ground. The difference is that your eyes stay focused straight ahead or slightly down.

Perform this drill in a series of rapid vertical jumps.

- Stand in an upright and balanced position.

- Quick drop to a quarter squat position—ankles, knees, hips, shoulders, and elbows are flexed.

- Immediately jump and simultaneously drive your knees to your elbows (arm-position is horizontal to the ground).

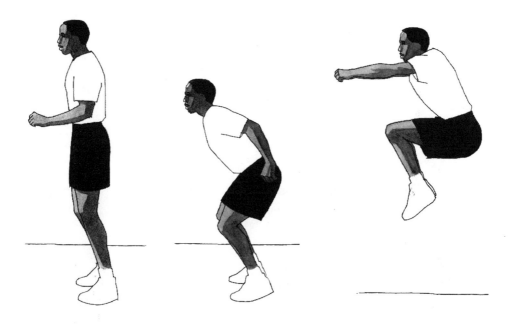

BARRIER JUMPS: FORWARD & BACK

By putting into play an obstacle like a small foam barrier, rolled-up towel, or collapsible hurdle, you now have a visual cue as to how high you need to jump.

You can vary the height of the barrier, use more than one such barrier, and alter the distance between barriers. Using a number of barriers will allow you to vary your stride length or jump length (for example, the barriers might be evenly spaced at 3-foot intervals).

For most plyometric exercises, emphasis is placed on the speed of the jump. This is particularly true with barrier jumps since the height of the jump is already known. As a result, you can focus on developing speed and quickness.

This is an excellent drill for improving your agility and foot speed; it requires only one barrier; after you've mastered one barrier, try the drill with 2 or 3 barriers.

- To begin, select a barrier that is 6 inches or less in height and width (as your technique and strength improve, you can increase the height of the barrier).

- Stand in a balanced, upright position, eyes focused on the approximate landing spot for your first jump.

- Keep your feet together, with your toes a couple of inches from the barrier.

- Slightly flex your shoulders and elbows so they are ready to assist in the jump. Don't let your arms drop from this position during the drill.

- Jump forward over the barrier. Jump far enough so your heels don't touch the barrier. Don't let your feet turn to one side (which is a common mistake); keep them pointing straight ahead.

- Immediately reverse the jump. Maintain your body control and jump backward to the initial starting position. Don't stop until you complete the set.

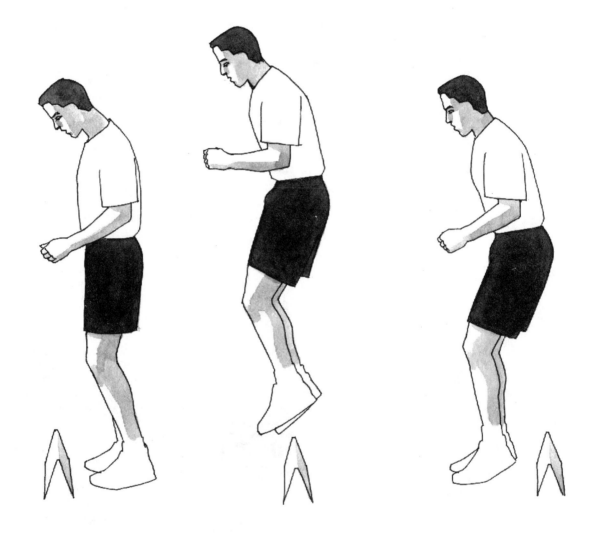

BARRIER JUMPS: SIDE TO SIDE

Basketball requires the ability to move laterally quickly, explosively, and efficiently. The following drill specifically trains the adductors and abductors of the legs, which are important muscles for lateral movement.

- To begin, select a barrier that is 6 inches or less in height and width (again, as technique and strength levels improve, you can increase the height of the barrier).

- Stand in an upright position, eyes focused on the approximate landing spot for your first jump.

- Place your feet together and parallel to the barrier. Your feet should be a comfortable distance from the side of the barrier. Remember, the barrier is at your side.

- Jump sideways over the barrier and land in the same "ready" position, ready for the next jump.

- Immediately repeat the jump in the opposite direction. Don't stop between side-to-side jumps until you complete the set.

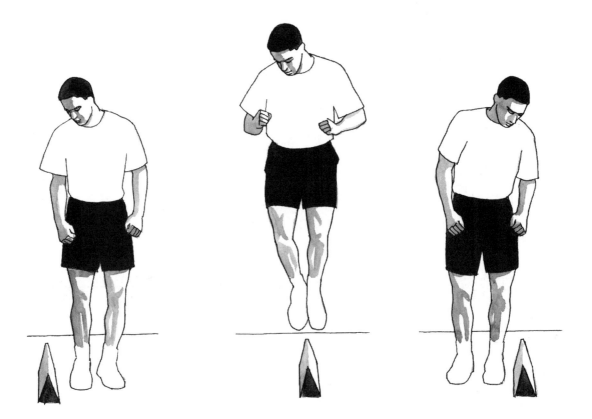

BOX JUMPS: UP & DOWN REPEATS—FORWARD

The next four drills will require a box approximately 9 to 12 inches in height. The best width for a box is 24 inches, and the length should be 36 inches. Box drills require you to raise your entire body weight the height of the box. More importantly, you must then be able to control the impact of your body weight when it is combined with the force of gravity upon landing (during every jump). As in all types of jumping, speed off the ground is critical.

• Stand on the box with your feet together. Your heels should be "hanging" over the edge.
• Slightly flex your shoulders and elbows so they are ready to assist in the jump. Don't let your arms drop from this position throughout the drill.
• Next, drop, don't jump, off the box.
• Upon contact with the ground, immediately jump back up to the starting position. Concentrate on quickness. Your heels shouldn't touch the ground.

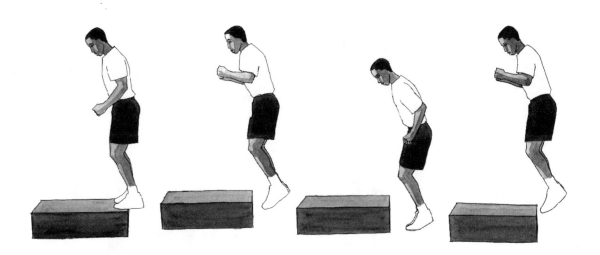

CONDITIONING TIP: If there's no box available, then a stair step would work just as well for this drill.

BOX JUMPS: UP & DOWN REPEATS—LATERAL

All professional basketball players know the importance of mastering explosive lateral movements.

They're a valuable asset to anyone at any level of athletic development.

This is an excellent drill for promoting lateral power.

- Stand on the box with your feet parallel to each other and close to the edge.

- Slightly flex your shoulders and elbows so they're ready to assist in the jump. Don't let your arms drop from this position throughout the drill.

- Now, drop laterally off the box. Make sure the drop is far enough away from the box to avoid catching your foot or ankle on the edge.

- When you reach the ground, immediately jump back up to your starting position. Concentrate on touch-and-go action with the ground. And realize that in many cases your heels will not touch down.

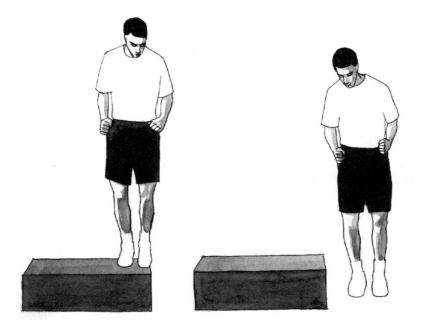

LATERAL BOX SHUFFLE

This is a tremendous drill for developing lateral movement and agility. This plyometric exercise works best when you use a short box (9 inches or less). Be sure to shuffle across the narrow width—24 inches—of the box.

- Stand next to the box with your outside foot on the floor and the other foot positioned on top and in the middle of the box.

- Focus your eyes on the box.

- Hold your arms in the defensive, "ready" position.

- Lift up slightly with the leg positioned on the box and quickly shift your weight across to the other side.

- Keep your center of gravity low.

- After crossing the box, your feet should make contact simultaneously, (that is to say, the "ground foot" and the "box foot" should land at the same time).

- Immediately repeat in the opposite direction.

- Speed is important, but safety is critical. Therefore, make sure your have enough clearance between your foot and the edge of the box. Don't perform this drill if you're tired.

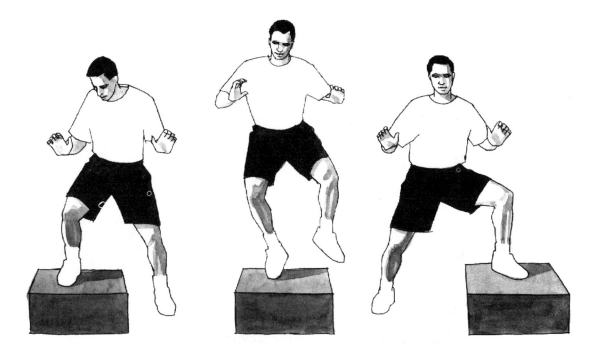

BOX DROP JUMP SHOT

This a great drill to develop vertical jump ability while at the same time performing a basketball skill such as catching and shooting. This exercise will certainly challenge your coordination, agility, and power.

- Position a box within your shooting range (that is to say, at the free-throw line, top of the key, etc.).

- Stand on the floor behind the box facing the basket.

- A coach or partner, holding a ball, positions himself between the box and the basket.

- Jump with both feet onto the box and quickly drop down to the floor on the other side.

- The ball is quickly passed sometime between the start of the first jump and the landing on the opposite side of the box.

- You should catch the ball prior to landing on the floor. Once you make contact with the floor, immediately and explosively jump as high as you can and shoot a jump shot.

- After the shot, the coach rebounds the ball while you prepare for the next repetition.

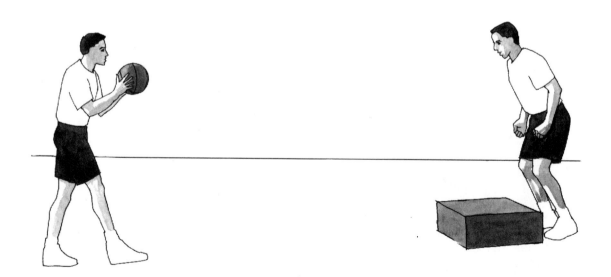

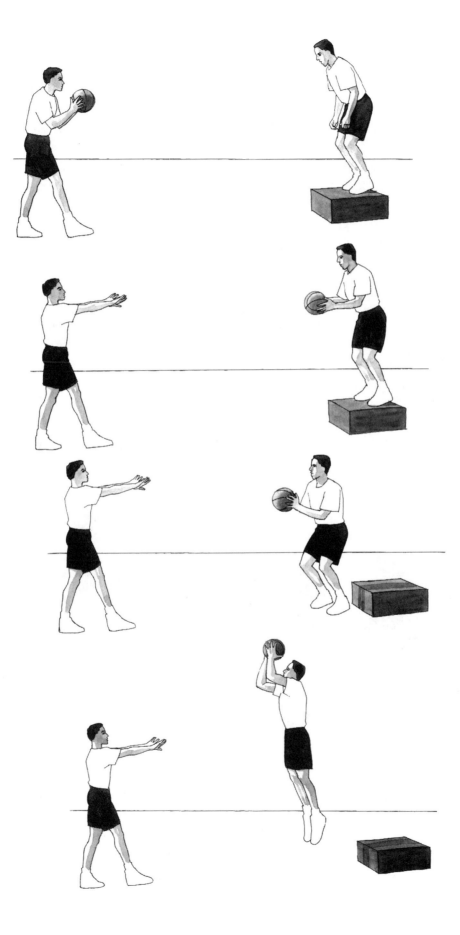

MEDICINE BALL TOSS

This drill can be done using either a single-arm toss (1- to 4-pound ball) or as a double-arm exercise (4- to 12-pound ball). This exercise is an example of a double-arm toss. The medicine ball toss develops power in your upper body.

- Stand 3 to 4 feet from a solid wall, feet shoulder-width apart.

- Grasp a rubber medicine ball on both sides. Now raise the ball over your head, with your elbows flexed to a 45-degree angle, and with your thumbs pointing down.

- Extend your elbows explosively, and the ball will fly hard against the wall. Be sure to aim slightly higher than the your hands at the point of the ball's release.

- When the ball rebounds back to you, your arms should be almost fully extended as you catch the ball. The momentum of the ball will drive your arms back to a position where the elbows are approximately at a 45-degree angle.

- Immediately repeat this process.

- Do 15 to 50 repetitions per set.

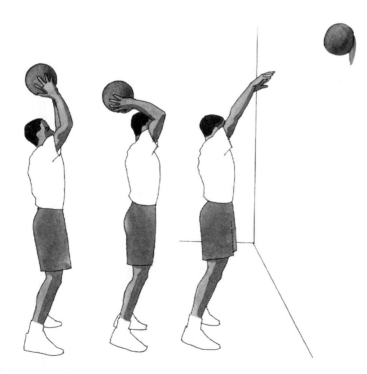

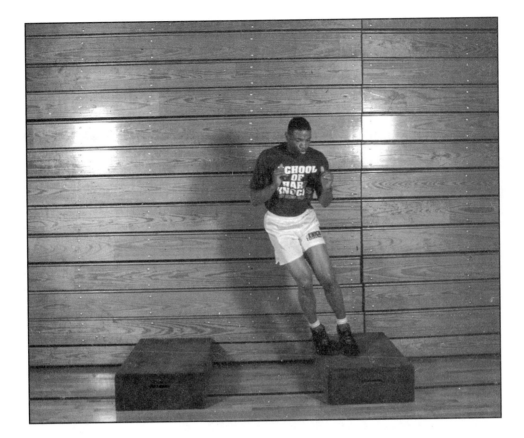

Doc Rivers of the **New York Knicks** is doing
lateral box jumps with two boxes.

MEDICINE BALL SQUAT TOSS

A 6- to 12-pound medicine ball works best for this drill. Make sure you can control a lighter ball before advancing to a heavier one. As with all medicine ball drills, make sure that you apply your best technique. For example, throw the ball with your legs and hips. Never "throw the ball with your back." When a drill is designed to develop leg power, then let your legs be the primary muscles performing the work. The Squat Toss is an excellent drill for developing power in your legs and shoulder girdle.

- First, stand in a balanced and upright position, with your feet slightly wider than shoulder width.
- Hold the ball at arms' length.

- Start by quickly dropping to a quarter squat position—with ankles, knees, and hips flexed. Arms remain straight during the drop. Keep your back straight and tight.
- Immediately drive your legs straight up as if jumping to the ceiling.
- Start the momentum of the ball with your legs, and continue the ball's movement by using your upper body and arms. At the instant you release the ball, your body should be fully extended.
- Toss the ball as high as possible. Avoid using your back to throw the ball. Concentrate on making your legs and shoulder girdle perform the toss. If done correctly, you can literally "jump into the throw."
- After the throw, do not catch the ball. Allow the ball to bounce off the ground and then use it for subsequent tosses.

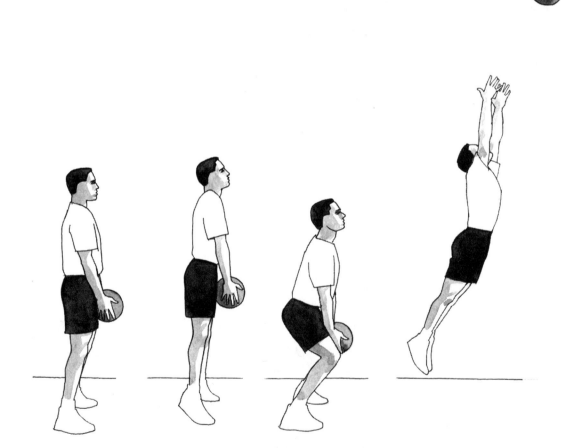

SPEED

Your speed is the time it takes you to move from point *A* to point *B,* running between 90 to 100% of your capacity. This may take 10 steps or 100 steps. You may dash from baseline to baseline or from one cone to another. It may be a 40-yard sprint or a 100-yard dash.

Simply put, the shorter the amount of time it takes you to move from one point to the next, the faster you are. The information and drills in this chapter are to help you develop the speed you already have.

The first thing you have to learn is that speed development, at least as far as basketball is concerned, isn't limited to sprinting straight ahead. On the court there are a lot of movement patterns that aren't straight forward:

- the defensive shuffle
- the backpedal
- change of direction

The second thing to notice is that the same principles involved in sprinting straight forward apply to these other movements.

What really determines your speed? Whether straight forward or straight backward, there are two basic components associated with speed:

- stride length—the distance covered in a single step; and,
- stride frequency—the number of steps taken in a given unit of time.

You reach your fastest sprinting form when you have a high rate of arm and leg frequency combined with a long stride. This is true for sprinters who want to run straight ahead as fast as possible, and it is true for athletes whose sport requires a high degree of lateral, backward, or combination movements.

As mentioned, speed is running between 90 to 100% of your capacity. But, remember our definition: Speed is the time it takes you to move from point *A* to point *B* or:

STRIDE FREQUENCY x STRIDE LENGTH = SPEED

You can improve your stride frequency and stride length by increasing the amount of force you produce from your legs. Stride frequency is accomplished by moving your arms and legs fast.

Naturally each individual has inherent limitations as to how fast he can move his arms and legs. Small gains in frequency can lead to tremendous success in the outcome of a race. More athletes can stand to improve their stride frequency, but the quicker dividend can be earned by developing an explosive stride length.

The following drills will help you attain that unique combination of skills.

SPEED MYTH

Many people believe that a person is born with speed and can't be taught to run faster. This is simply not true.

Athletes can be trained to sprint faster, just like singers can be taught to sing better. While you may not be genetically blessed to run as fast as Carl Lewis, you can certainly make a significant improvement in your present speed.

Sprinting is considered by many coaches to be the most fundamental of all athletic movements. In order to improve your sprinting performance you must become familiar with the technical elements involved with the movement.

It may be true that some athletes have a greater potential for improvement than others. But the key is to recognize that most athletes have not fully realized their sprinting potential.

We ask that you spend some time studying and practicing the techniques taught in this chapter. Why? Because, with practice, the sprinting techniques you learn here will stay with you throughout your competitive years.

SPEED WORKOUT

Athletes like **Kevin Johnson**, **Tim Hardaway**, and **Muggsy Bogues** make their movements on the court look smooth, effortless, and explosive. If your goal is to develop just as efficient and explosive a stride as theirs, you can do it.

You can do it by breaking the sprint action down into its parts and by practicing each part. Then when you reassemble the parts, your sprinting action will have greatly improved. In other words, by practicing each part of the whole movement, you'll be able to enhance your strengths and eliminate your weaknesses.

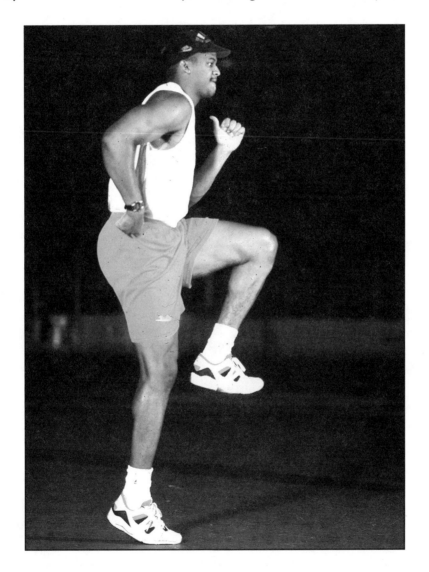

Labradford Smith of the **Sacramento Kings** is doing a marching exercise that develops knee lift for sprinting.

ARM MOVEMENT EXERCISES

An excellent way to begin working on arm movements is to be aware that your shoulder is a ball and socket joint. Consciously relax the muscles surrounding your shoulder. (You can tell your shoulders are relaxed when they "let go" toward the ground, rather than inch up toward the sky.) Maintain this relaxation throughout the exercise. Now move your arms slowly in a circle. The circular movement will help you feel and understand more about your shoulder's movement capabilities.

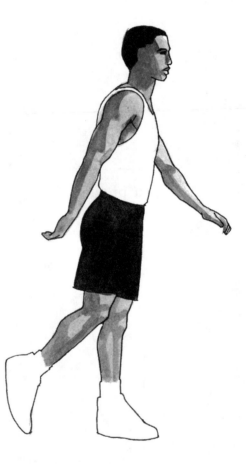

- First phase—swing your arms back and forth.

- Swing your arms in line with your forward motion. Emphasis should be placed on maintaining relaxed shoulders while you swing your arms straight forward and back.

- Second, let your hands and fingers be loose and relaxed like your shoulders. Clenching your fists will create tension in your forearms and shoulders and will then inhibit a free swinging movement at your shoulders.

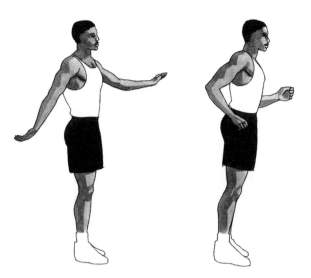

- The third phase involves bending your elbows to 90 degrees and again, allowing them to swing freely from the shoulder.

- Arms move forward and back.

- Never raise your arms higher than your chest or shoulder.

CONDITIONING TIP: As you progress in your practice, you can work on moving your arms faster while standing in place. Remember arm speed governs your leg speed. Make sure your hands and shoulders stay relaxed.

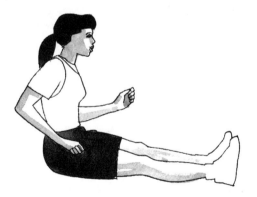

- Sit on the floor or on a bench with your legs extended.

- Pump your arms as if you were hitting down on an imaginary bongo drum.

THE ABC'S OF RUNNING

The running stride can be broken down into three phases—knee lift, leg reach, and back leg extension or push-off. Back leg extension or push-off is defined as the synergized extension of the hip, knee and ankle joints involving the gluteals, hamstrings and gastrocnemius.

Knee lift exercises will be referred to as category *A*, leg reach will be referred to as category *B*, and category *C* will refer to back leg extension (bounding).

EXERCISE A1

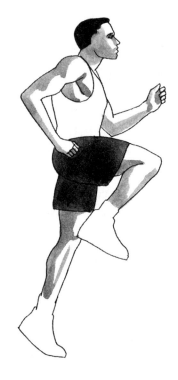

- March with the knees coming high and then down.

- Emphasize staying on the balls of the feet and maintain a straight body alignment while your knee drives "up."

- Keep your thigh parallel to the ground while the opposite leg stays straight.

- When your drive knee reaches its highest point (for example, thigh parallel to the ground), the ankle of the same leg should be plantar-flexed with the foot positioned directly under your knee.

EXERCISE A2

• Repeat exercise A1, except instead of marching, skip as you alternate legs.

EXERCISE **A3**

The final stage for knee lift work. This drill is similar to running, however you should really emphasize knee lift.

• During this drill, your stride length is limited.

• As you progress down the court or field, take approximately three steps per yard.

• Emphasize proper body alignment with the hips positioned under your torso. This will help to ease you into a full range of motion and allow for a more explosive stride due to a leverage advantage.

CONDITIONING TIP: A good way to work on body alignment is to keep your upper body in front of your belly button.

Exercises for the leg reach phase fall into Category *B*.

EXERCISE B1

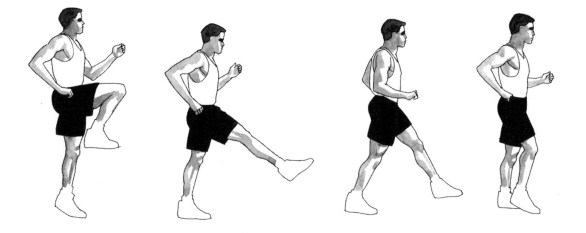

- Walk so as to drive the lead knee "up" and extend the leg at the knee joint.
- Pull back on the ground—the harder you pull back on the ground the harder the ground will push back against your force.

The back pulling action is important to insure that the foot does not make contact with the ground too far in advance of the body. Pulling will also alleviate any undesirable vertical body position. A good self-coaching cue is to continually reinforce the action of "leading with the knee" before extending your leg during the leg reach.

EXERCISE B2

- Include a skip between alternating legs.

EXERCISE **B3**

- Emphasize high knee lift, a good leg reach, and explosive gluteal and hamstring involvement (pulling back on the ground).

- Movement down the court or the field should be slow. Maintain proper body alignment, with your chest slightly in front of your body's center of gravity.

- Contact with the ground should be on the balls of your feet, not flat-footed.

CONDITIONING TIP: The ability to execute an explosive knee drive combined with an efficient leg reach will promote the development of a longer stride. The harder you pull back on the floor the harder the floor pushes back in the same direction you are pulling.

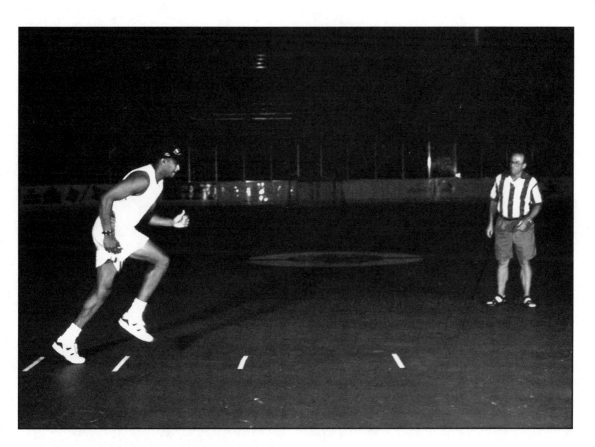

Al Biancani, Strength and Conditioning Coach of the **Sacramento Kings,** is having **Labradford Smith** work on a stride length exercise.

Category *C* is the third phase of the stride and consists of the back leg extension or "push."

EXERCISE C1

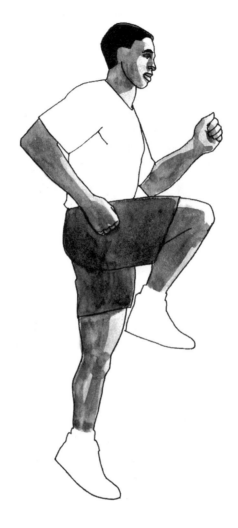

- This is a hopping drill, following hop pattern: RIGHT—RIGHT; LEFT— LEFT; RIGHT—RIGHT; and so on.

- Focus on a full extension of the back leg, and on attaining as much height as possible.

- Similar to the A exercises, the lead leg is brought up, the emphasis is skipping high in the air extending the other leg and pushing up and back.

- Distance on the hop is not as important as performing correct technique.

EXERCISE C2

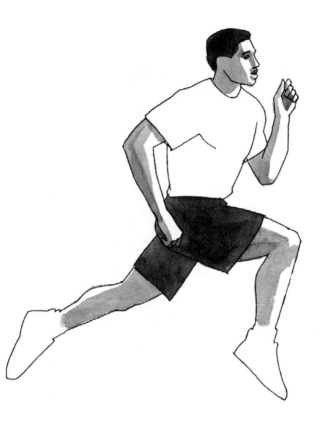

- This exaggerated form of sprinting is called bounding.

- Emphasis is on developing a full extension of the back or "push" leg. Unlike the hopping drill, you alternate the leg action: RIGHT—LEFT—RIGHT.

- During the knee drive phase there is a slight pause. It's during this hesitation that you'll be in flight. You should stress full extension of the hip and knee, and plantar-flexion of the ankle, during the "push."

- You should try to get as much distance as possible between bounds. This will force you to really extend your back leg.

CONDITIONING TIP: As with all drills up to this point, you must maintain proper arm action at all times. And you must maintain a position high on the balls of your feet. Foot and ankle strength are vitally important for developing an explosive push-off.

ANKLE FLIPS

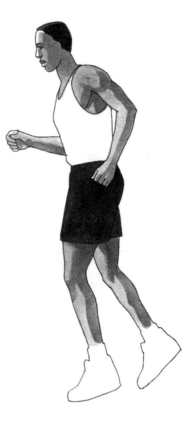

- Get as high on the balls of the feet as possible, "flop" the feet as you step forward.

- Forcefully point your toes in alternating fashion.

- Knees should be slightly bent.

- As the right foot pushes off the left foot should slide along the floor surface.

- Be sure to land on your toes and not flat-footed.

CONDITIONING TIP: Just before you are about to take a step, note the position of your body. You should be in perfect alignment (shoulder, hip, knee, and ankle are in a straight line), with your chest in advance of your center of gravity. Maintain this perfect body position, as you begin this drill. This will give you a feeling of being tall while you are running.

4-STEP ACCELERATION DRILL

We have discussed, at some detail, how to sprint properly. Now let's focus on developing your ability to accelerate.

The ability to get your body moving from a standstill to a full sprint in the shortest possible time cannot be overemphasized in the game of basketball. The following exercises sequence is to help develop your ability to accelerate.

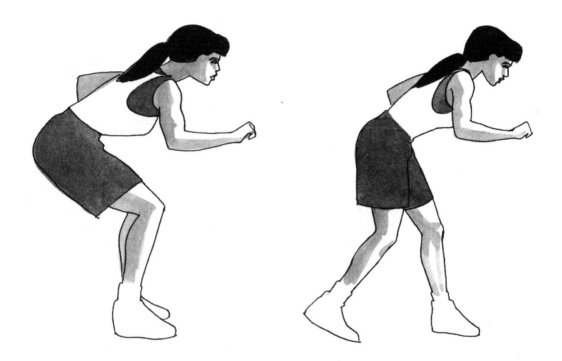

- Stand and punch arms.

- Then punch your arms and take a step.

- Punch your arms and take a short step.

- Try to punch the lead arm parallel to the ground; this will help eliminate any tendency to shift the body into the unwanted vertical position.

- Emphasize moving your arms quickly and "beating down on your hip" (like the bongo drum).

- Mark the distance. Put tape or some sort of marker on the floor to serve as a visual cue that will help dictate your quick stride length.

- The recommended distance is 28" for step one, 38" between step 1 and 2, 48" between step 2 and 3, and 58" between steps 3 and 4.

- The distances are not what your normal stride length will be when you are at top speed. The taped distances are used as a pattern to get your feet down so you can get to top speed quickly. (These distances are based on the average steps of an adult basketball player; you may have to adjust them downward to suit your age and size.)

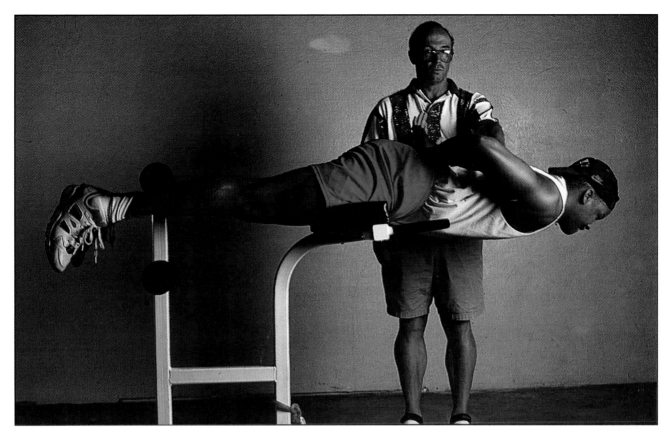

Al Biancani, strength and conditioning coach of the Sacramento Kings observes Labradford Smith doing a back extension.

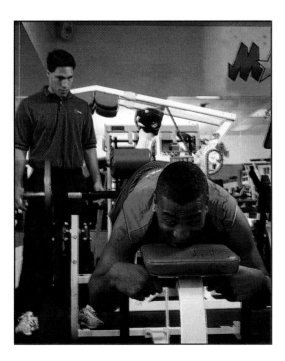

David Oliver, strength and conditioning coach of the Orlando Magic observes Dennis Scott working on the leg curl machine.

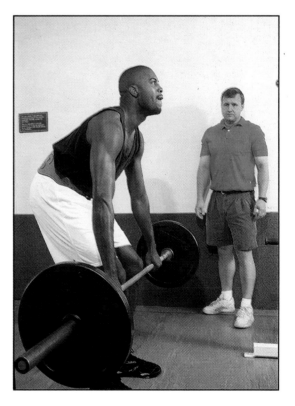

Bill Foran, strength and conditioning coach of the Miami Heat observes Glen Rice, who is ready to perform a hang clean.

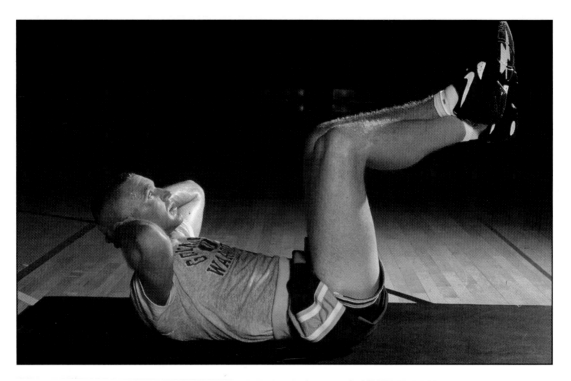

All-Star Chris Mullin of the Golden State Warriors and the original Dream Team is doing an abdominal crunch.

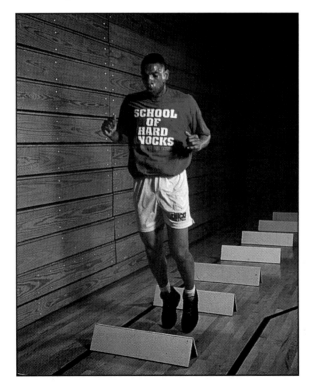

Doc Rivers of the New York Knicks is doing a plyometric jumping drill over barriers.

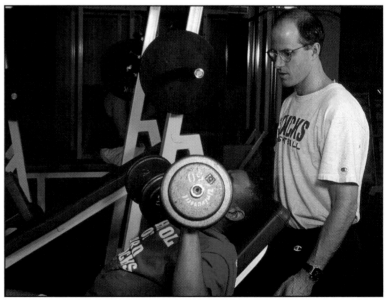

Greg Brittenham, strength and conditioning coach of the New York Knicks spots Doc Rivers on the dumbbell incline press.

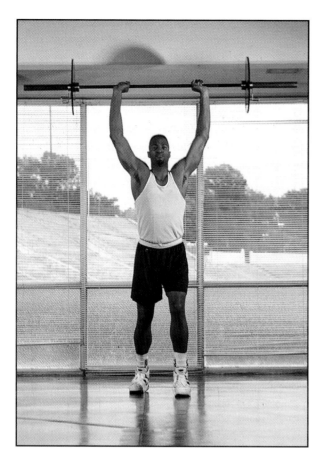

All-Star center and Dream Team II member
Alonzo Mourning of the Charlotte Hornets is
doing a standing military press.

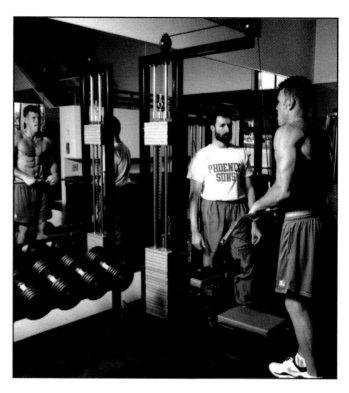

Robin Pound, strength and conditioning coach
of the Phoenix Sun watches Dan Majerle,
All-Star guard and member of Dream Team II
perform the tricep press down.

Bob King strength and conditioning coach of
the Dallas Mavericks is working out Greg
Drieling on a plyometric jumping device.

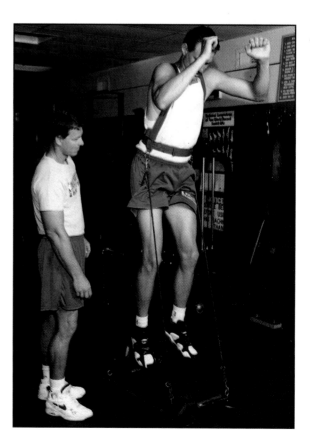

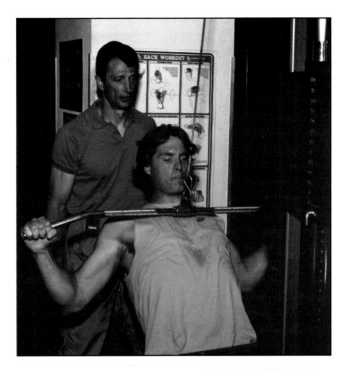

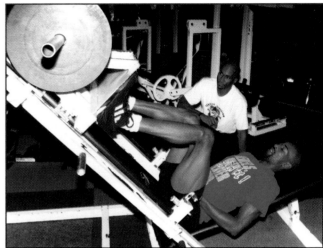

Sol Brandys, strength and conditioning coach of the Minnesota Timberwolves spots Christian Laetner on the lat pulldown.

Roger Hinds, strength and conditioning coach of the Atlanta Hawks watches as Stacey Augmon works out the leg press.

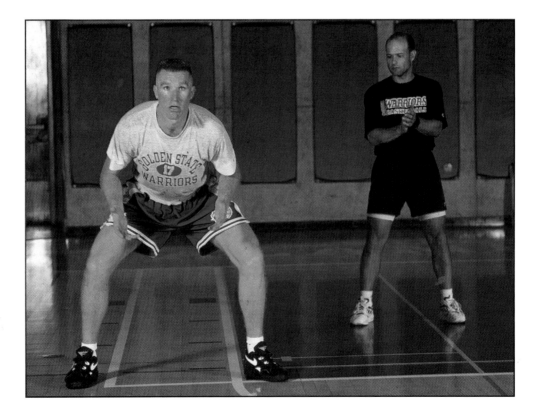

Mark Grabow, strength and conditioning coach of the Golden State Warriors has Chris Mullin doing the lateral slide with response drill.

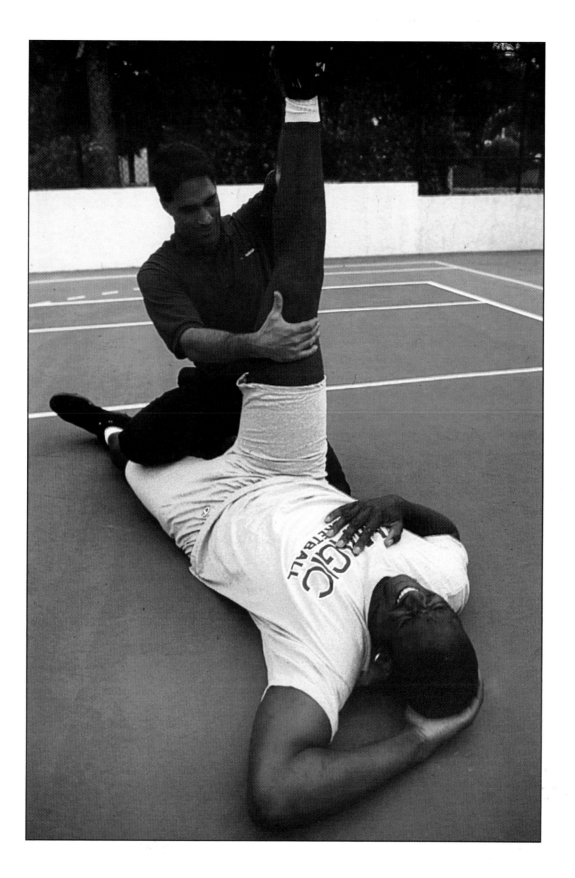

Dave Oliver stretching All-Star Center and Dream Team II member
Shaquille O'Neal.

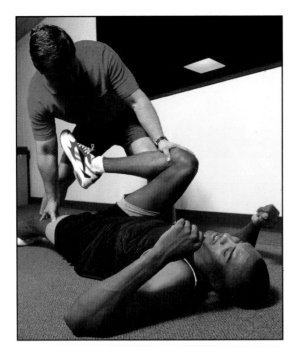

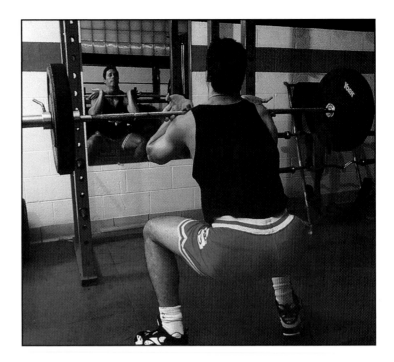

Bill Foran is stretching Steve Smith's low back. Steve was a member of Dream Team II.

Tom Gugliotta of the Washington Bullets shows excellent technique with the front squat.

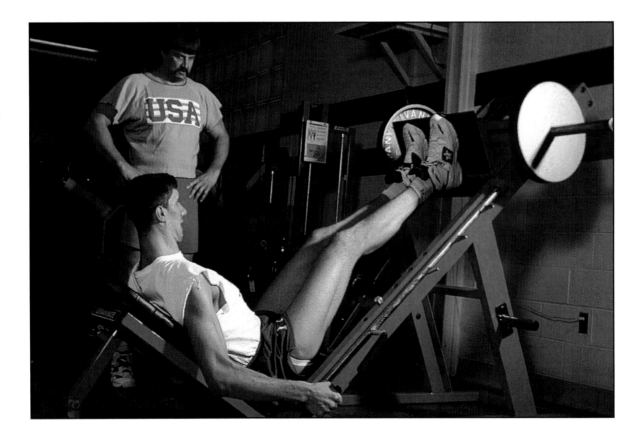

Strength and conditioning coach Dennis Householder is monitoring Washington Bullets center, 7' 7" Gheorge Muresan working out on the leg press.

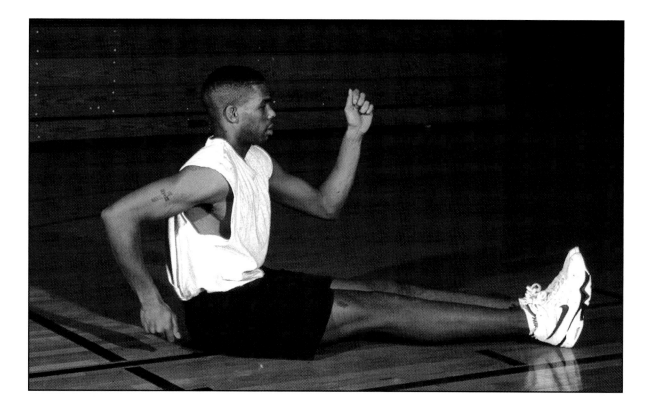

Hubert Davis of the New York Knicks is doing a seated arm movement
exercise for his speed development.

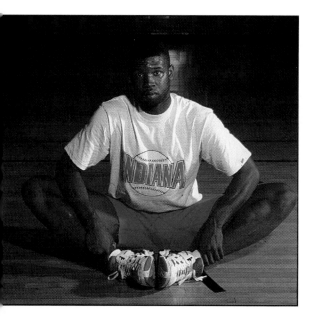

Calbert Cheaney of the Washington Bullets is
doing an individual static stretch of the groin.

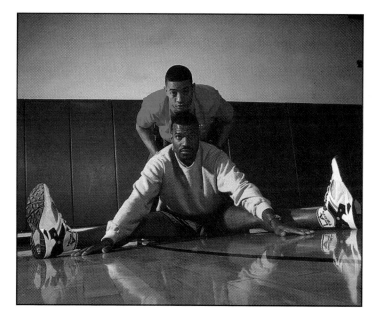

Carl Horne, strength and conditioning coach of
the Los Angeles Clippers is stretching
Loy Vaught.

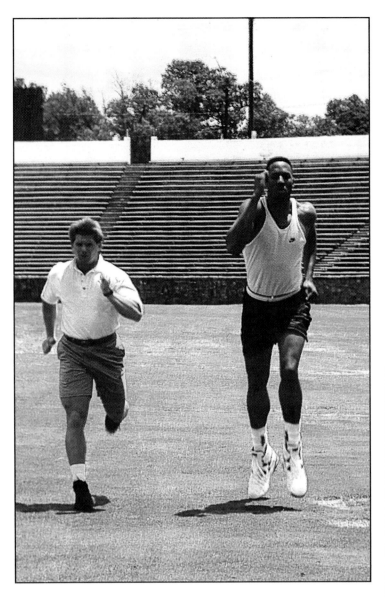

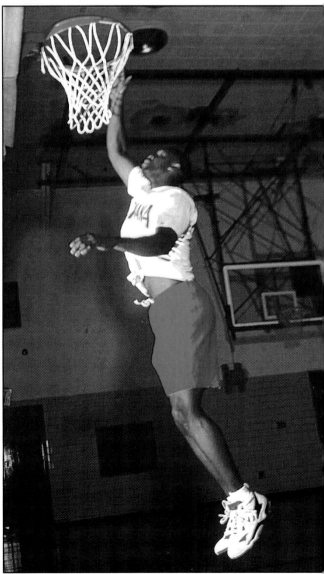

Chip Sigmon, strength and conditioning coach of the Charlotte Hornets conditions Alonzo Mourning.

Calbert Cheaney of Washington Bullets is performing "rim jumps," a plyometric exercise.

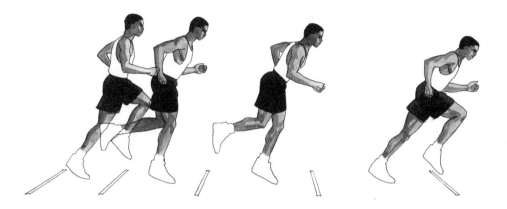

- Use the lines you have marked and start going through the 4- steps at $1/4$ effort.

- Emphasis should be on getting your lead arm back on your hip to avoid any hesitation between the first and second step.

- Make forceful moves, the more forceful you beat down on your hip, the more powerfully your opposite leg will drive.

Once you become proficient with the technique at $1/4$ speed, you can graduate to $1/2$ effort, $3/4$ effort, and then all out effort.

After you learn to do the 4-step drill from a line, then face the basket, turn and start toward the other basket using the 4-step concept.

Other drills can include: changing from a backpedal to a sprint with an emphasis on the first 4 steps, or going from a defensive position into a sprint using the same concept.

BEGINNING A SPRINT

- Stand up straight, with your shoulders, knees, hips, and ankles properly aligned.

- During the power phase of a sprint, your foot exerts a powerful "push" force to the ground, propelling your body forward.

- As you begin running, your body will automatically shift into a slightly forward lean. Remember to keep your upper body in front of your belly button.

To insure proper sprinting technique, you must achieve total balance and coordinate your limbs in a synchronized rhythm. Remember sprinting is a rhythmic losing and gaining of your balance.

Adhere to the following checklist to fully maximize your sprint potential:

1. Body alignment is critical. Your ear, shoulder, hip, knee, and ankle should be in a straight line. This position should be maintained when you're sprinting and through the duration of the drills.

2. Your shoulders should be squared and relaxed, with no torso rotation.

3. Keep your elbows at a 90° angle. Don't let your angle change. Keep your elbows in, swinging close to your body.

4. Keep your hands slightly open. They should go no higher than your shoulders on the forward swing and no further back than your hips on the back swing.

5. Fully extend your push leg (but do not overextend as that will cause you to fall out of balance and rhythm).

6. Drive the knee of your drive leg in a straight line forward, not upward.

7. Keep your eyes focused straight ahead. Avoid head movement up, down, or to the side.

Apply the principles you have learned in this chapter with the sprinting program in the conditioning chapter. Proper mechanics and running form are vital to making the most of your speed and stamina. It requires patience to ultimately realize physical changes. In time, you'll definitely see improvement in the speed of your movements.

These drills emphasize actual sprint technique, but please remember that these very same principles apply to other movements such as shuffling, backpedaling, defensive slides, and many other combinations that basketball players will certainly use during the course of a game.

To help you keep a record of your work, place a check mark in the appropriate column on the chart as you complete the drills. Do not do the Sprinting Program in the Conditioning Chapter until you have filled in the Speed Drill Chart. Make sure you warm up before you start exercising and cool down when you finish exercising.

SPEED DRILL CHART

Exercise	Date	Date	Date	Date	Date	Date	Date	Date
Arm Movement								
Running Stride: A 1								
A 2								
A 3								
B 1								
B 2								
B 3								
C 1								
C 2								
Ankle Flips								
4-Step Acceleration								
Beginning a Sprint								

WEIGHT-TRAINING

Many young athletes are eager to train, but do not know how to train properly. This is partly due to the vast amounts of misinformation in the strength-training field. A properly designed functional weight training program for basketball increases performance and reduces the chances of injuries. This performance is enhanced by increases in strength, speed, power, and flexibility. The confidence gained from these improvements in your play may take your game to the next level.

This chapter is designed in proper sequence. Follow this sequence to fully understand the total program. Dedicated basketball players, coaches, and perhaps parents may all benefit from this information.

"Weight-training has helped me mentally and physically," says **Anfernee "Penny" Hardaway** of the **Orlando Magic**. "Knowing I've increased my strength not only increases my confidence but also helps my defensive and offensive performance."

"Weight-training gives me the strength to make it through the long and grinding NBA season averaging over 40 minutes a game," says **Dan Majerle** of the **Phoenix Suns**. "It helps me perform and maintain higher levels of intensity while reducing my chances of injury."

"Weight-training," says **Kevin Johnson** of the **Phoenix Suns**, "helps give me the power and durability to consistently penetrate and challenge the NBA's best big men night after night."

INTRODUCTION TO TECHNICAL INFORMATION

This section, along with the Appendices (pages 226-233), has all the information you need to fully understand the weight-training programs and how to use them properly and safely for the best results.

Practical information and weight-room safety considerations.

A. Determining the amount of weight for an exercise.

B. Trial-and-error method

C. Breathing

D. Wearing a belt

E. Adequate spacing

F. Proper balance of weight on the bar

G. Spotting

H. Lift-off and return

I. Speed of movement

J. Rest periods

K. Exercise order

L. Exercise techniques: illustrations and explanations

WEIGHT-ROOM SAFETY

HOW MUCH WEIGHT?

How much weight should you use when performing an exercise? Either you can follow the traditional trial-and-error method, use a percentage of body weight, or you can follow a more scientific approach by using percentages of your own strength.

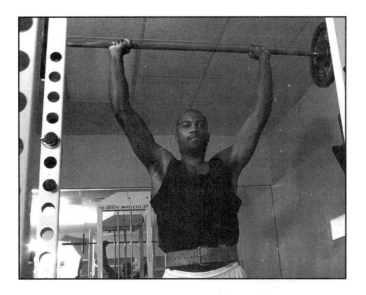

Glen Rice of the **Miami Heat** is doing a standing military press.

We have decided to present the trial-and-error procedure.

When you start an exercise routine, you must do three things:

1. warm-up with a light weight to prevent injury in the affected muscular area performing the work;

2. choose a comfortable weight for the first set of the exercise without straining; and

3. progressively increase the weight to become stronger and better conditioned.

TRIAL AND ERROR

In the beginning of your weight-training program, you can establish your true training-resistance for each exercise. Simply choose a light, comfortable weight to begin the exercise. Then make the weight heavier until you can feel the amount of resistance that is needed to perform the exercise correctly for a desired number of repetitions. Once this weight is established, you now have a general idea of your training-resistance for this particular exercise.

BREATHING

There are three simple rules to remember about breathing.

1. Always breathe.

2. Breathe out (exhale) during the most difficult phase of the exercise; for example, raising the bar during an arm curl.

3. Breathe in (inhale) during the easiest phase of the exercise; for example, lowering the bar during the arm curl.

It's probably a good idea to inhale before starting the movement, to hold the breath during the beginning of the movement, and to exhale when two-thirds of the exercise is completed. This method of breathing will allow for a large blood return to the heart, and thus reduce heart distress. If an individual holds his breath throughout the entire exercise, such cardiac problems as elevated blood pressure and irregular heartbeats may occur.

If an individual doesn't breathe properly when exerting effort, especially during weight-training, a symptom known as the "Valsalva effect" may result. This term describes a rise in blood pressure during which fainting or dizziness may occur.

However, there are exceptions to these rules of breathing for the explosive, Olympic-type movements. When performing the power clean, the exhalation of air comes after the squat-and-catch phase, and before the ascent. During the ascent, the lifter may produce short inhalations followed by short exhalations.

WEARING A BELT

A weight-lifting belt provides added support to the muscles surrounding the lower spine. The abdominal muscles in particular are aided by using a belt; it gives them something to push against when performing a high-effort, maximum or sub-maximum, multi-joint exercise, like a squat.

SPACE

Be sure you have enough space to perform your exercise. Are there any weights (dumbbells, bars, or plates) in or around your area of training? Is the floor dry for proper footing? Are there any pieces of rubberized flooring or carpet overlapping? Do you have enough space between exercise machines to move around without bumping into anything?

PROPER BALANCE OF WEIGHT ON THE BAR

Before you start to lift any weights take a couple of seconds to ask yourself a few questions.

1. Is the weight the same on both sides?
2. Are the collars on both sides?
3. Are the collars securely fastened?

SPOTTING

Spot is the term applied when asking for assistance in training, for example, "Excuse me, can you give me a spot?" Spotting is the act of observing and/or physically helping an individual through an exercise. "Physically helping" means assisting in raising the weight or aiding in the balancing process when the lifter performs an exercise (body or weight).

The spotter can spot either by using a lot of assistance or by barely helping the lifter throughout the movement, whichever the person needs or wants.

When you are the spotter, be sure to keep your eyes on the bar and the position of the lifter's body at all times. Look for a breakdown in technique, for a loss of balance, a "sticking point" (no movement) during the exercise, or for a bar moving out of the proper exercise groove.

INITIAL LIFT-OFF AND RETURN

Exercises such as the bench press and the seated shoulder press may require a lift-off to start the movement. There is a correct way to do this. Again, this is a personal thing.

The most common procedure in a lift-off is as follows:

1. The spotter or lifter counts to three.
2. On three, the spotter and the lifter, together, lift the weight to the starting position.
3. Once the lifter has the weight stable by himself, the spotter removes his hands from the bar or weight.
4. Then the lifter lowers the weight to begin the exercise.

Usually, the spotter's hands are spaced evenly along the bar, with one hand over the bar while the other hand is placed underneath the bar. This allows for a well-balanced and well-controlled lift-off. The spotter helps the lifter both out of and back into the rack.

SPEED OF MOVEMENT

Control both the lowering and raising phases of the lift. Each repetition should be performed with a smooth, controlled movement. However, when performing explosive movements, each repetition is completed as fast as possible with proper technique.

REST PERIODS

Rest periods play a major role in establishing each muscle's potential strength or endurance level. The longer the rest period between each working set, the more time a muscle has to replenish its energy supply. Therefore, the muscle has a greater potential of becoming stronger.

Conversely, a shorter rest period (say, 30 to 90 seconds) will allow for an increase in potential endurance levels, while causing a decrease in potential strength levels. These two factors must be taken into consideration when prescribing rest periods for resistance training.

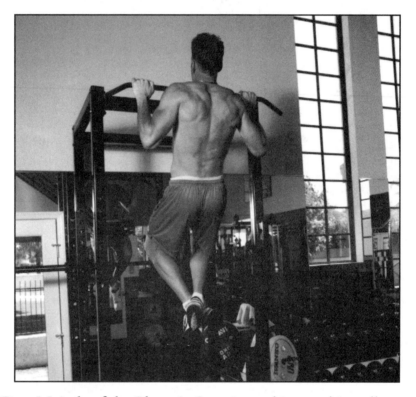

Dan Majerle of the **Phoenix Suns** is working on his pull-ups.

LONGER REST PERIODS

Don't wait until your body has cooled down between sets before you begin to perform the next set. Such a delay increases the chance of injuries; your body has to handle heavy weight when it's no longer fully prepared. In most cases, 3 to 5 minutes is enough of a rest period.

EXERCISE ORDER

In general, you should work the larger major muscle-group exercises first, then work your way to the smaller muscle-group exercises.

If you do a total body program in the same day, split your body in half, and follow this philosophy for both upper-body and lower-body exercises. Some people have target body parts and/or exercises that they want to do first or pre-fatigue before doing the rest of the program. In these special cases, you may do these exercises first.

EXERCISE ILLUSTRATIONS AND TECHNIQUES

This section contains a number of exercises, with an illustration and brief explanation for each to show the correct and the safe technique.

Following this section are three weight-training programs.

Some cautions: No two people are exactly alike. There are individual differences that you need to be aware of as they relate to the proper technique of weight-training exercises. The first thing you should do on a given exercise is to adjust the equipment and weight to fit your body and individual needs. Very few people are capable of perfect technique on all lifts. Technique may vary depending on individual differences. Adjustments in range of motion, grips, stances, and grooves may have to be made. To be on the safe side, have a qualified coach or instructor evaluate your lifting technique.

Again, just to be safe, when you're the spotter in a dumbbell exercise and you see the dumbbells straying from the proper exercise groove, grab the wrists of the lifter so that you can help guide the dumbbells back into the proper groove.

ABDOMINAL PROGRAM

Why develop the abdominals? Abdominal strength is essential to the athlete because it helps protect the body from injury, notably to the lower-back area. It also helps create greater stability throughout the mid-section and aids the spinal erectors in postural alignments of the vertebral column and pelvis. Greater abdominal and hip flexor strength may also increase running speed, stamina, and knee-lift.

We have evaluated many different abdominal programs and, in so doing, have developed an abdominal program that we feel provides both abdominal strength and endurance by using only the safest and most effective exercises.

DICTIONARY OF EXERCISE TERMS

The following is a list of terms that you will need to know in order to understand the exercises and programs below.

Hip flexors: the hip flexors raise the legs toward the chest when the upper body is fixed, and move the chest toward the legs when they are fixed.

Flexors of the spine: the rectus abdominus and internal/external obliques all flex or curl the spine.

Rotators of the spine: the rectus abdominus, internal/external obliques, semispinalis, multifidus, rotatores and levatores muscles all contribute to the rotation of the spine.

Prime mover: the primary muscle(s) involved in the movement.

Assistor: the assistor aids the prime movers with the movement.

Stabilizer: usually a muscle in a non-moving, isometric contraction stabilizing one body part so another body part, usually involving a prime mover, has something to pull against.

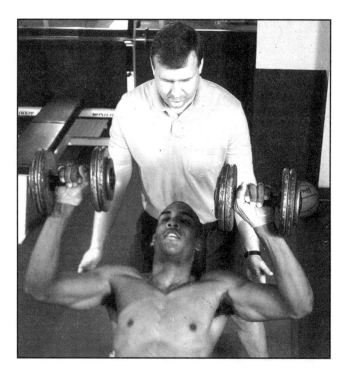

Bill Foran, Miami Heat's strength and conditioning coach is spotting **Steve Smith** as he performs a dumbbell incline press. **Steve** is now with the **Atlanta Hawks.**

BENT LEG RAISES

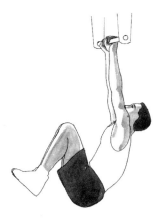

- Take a slightly wider-than-shoulder-width grip on a chin-up bar and keep your upper torso as relaxed as possible.

- Raise your knees all the way to your chest each time.

- The more your curl you spine at the top of the movement, the greater abdominal involvement you will have.

PRIME MOVER: hip flexors
STABILIZERS: abdominals and obliques

STRAIGHT LEG RAISES

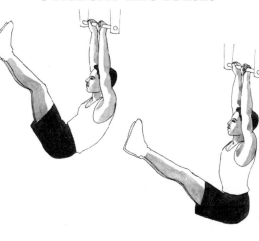

Correct position   Wrong position

- Take a slightly wider-than-shoulder-width grip on a chin-up bar and keep your upper torso as relaxed as possible.

- Raise your legs until your feet touch the bar.

- Your pelvis should rock forward as you raise your legs. This guarantees maximum abdominal involvement.

- Hold for a second or so, then lower legs back to the starting position.

Note: It's important that you lower your legs slowly enough so you don't start swinging; knees should be slightly bent throughout the exercise.

PRIME MOVER: hip flexors
STABILIZERS: abdominals and obliques

PRAYER CRUNCHES (FEET DOWN)

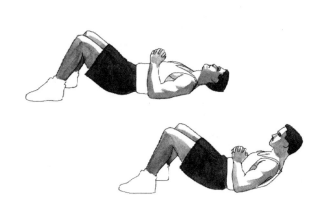

- Lie in the standard bent-leg sit-up position, and, raise your shoulders and upper back about 30-45 degrees off the ground.

- In this position your lower back should be flat against the ground.

- Hold for a second or so, then slowly return to starting position.

- Keep your arms in place but as relaxed as possible throughout exercise.

PRIME MOVERS: abdominals and obliques
STABILIZER: hip flexors

ROTARY CRUNCHES (FEET UP)

- Start in bent-knee sit-up position, both legs up off the floor, so both your hips and your knees form right angles.

- Place both hands behind your head.

- Raise shoulders 12 to 18 inches off the ground, turn your right elbow toward left knee, return to the ground, then raise up and rotate left elbow to right knee. (Counts as one repetition.)

PRIME MOVERS: rectus abdominis, internal/external obliques, semispinalis, multifidus, rotatores and levatores muscles; all contribute to rotation of the spine
STABILIZER: hip flexors

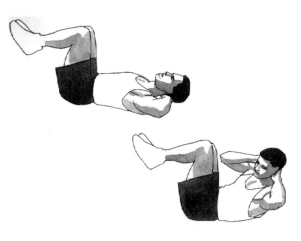

Perform these repetitions as rapidly as possible.

STRAIGHT LEG CRUNCHES

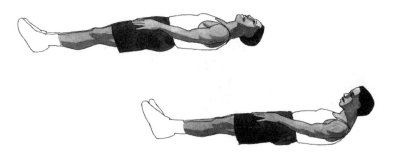

- Lie on your back, with legs straight out and hands on your thighs, palms down.

- Flex your abdominals, lift your shoulders slightly off the ground, and slide your hands down your thighs. Hold for a count then return.

- Your lower back should be flat against the ground in the flexed position.

PRIME MOVERS: abdominals and obliques
STABILIZER: hip flexors

ROTARY CRUNCHES (FEET DOWN)

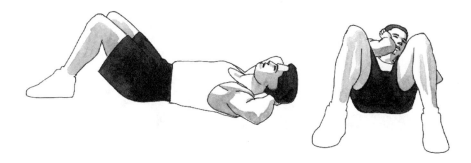

- These are a lot harder than previous exercises.

- Lie in bent-knee sit-up position, and slowly raise your shoulders and upper back off the ground.

- Your right elbow should turn toward (but not touch) your left knee.

- Hold at peak for at least one second, then slowly return to starting position, and repeat with left elbow turning toward the right knee.

PRIME MOVERS: rectus abdominis, internal/external obliques, semispinalis, multifidus, rotatores and levatores muscles all contribute to rotation of the spine
STABILIZER: hip flexors

CRUNCHES (FEET UP)

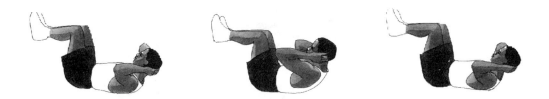

- Start in bent knee position with legs off the floor.

- Quickly raise upper back and shoulders off the floor, then lower and repeat.

- You should do these as fast as you can. Don't pull against neck or flap elbows; use abdominals.

PRIME MOVERS: abdominals and obliques
STABILIZER: hip flexors

QUICK TOUCHES (STRAIGHT LEGS)

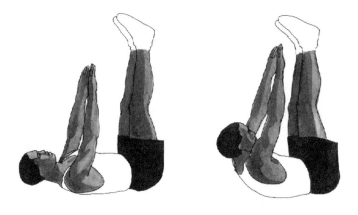

- Lie on the floor with your back down and legs straight up.

- Keeping legs straight, reach up and touch toes as quickly as possible.

- Don't completely return back flat to the ground in between repetitions.

PRIME MOVERS: abdominals and obliques
STABILIZER: hip flexors (in isometric contraction)

CONDITIONING TIP: Breathe normally, don't hold your breath.

KNEE ROCK BACKS

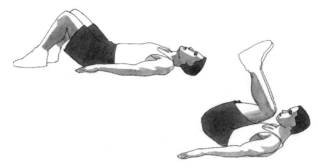

- Begin in bent-knee sit-up position, feet on the floor, but arms extended a few inches from your sides, palms down.

- Rock back until your knee hits your chest and your lower back comes off the floor.

- Lower and repeat.

- Curl your spine at the top of the movement to activate your abdominals to a greater extent.

PRIME MOVER: hip flexors
STABILIZERS: abdominal and obliques

LYING 6 " LEG RAISES

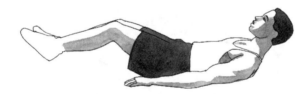

- Lie on your back, place hands, palms down, under pelvis. Your hands and arms should function as a cradle to prevent your back from arching.

- Keep your head and shoulders up with abdominals flexed to flatten your lower back against the ground. This limits the strain on the lower back.

- Raise the legs about 18"off the floor; then lower to about 12". Repeat up to 18" down to 12".

PRIME MOVER: hip flexors
STABILIZERS: abdominals and obliques

Note: If you feel pain in your lower back your abdominals may not yet be strong enough to do this exercise so skip it for a while until your abdominals are strengthened sufficiently.

STRAIGHT-UPS

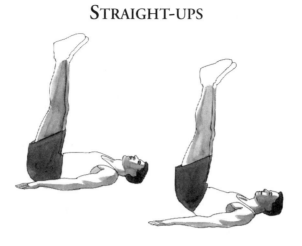

- Lie flat on your back with your arms at your sides for support. Legs should be together and straight up vertical to the ground.
- Raise legs and hips approximately 6 to 8 inches straight up, return to ground briefly, then repeat

PRIME MOVERS: abdominals and obliques
STABILIZER: hip flexors

SIDE-UPS

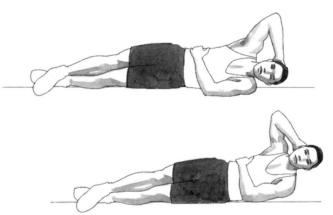

- Lie on your left side, left hand on right obliques, right hand on side of head.
- Legs are straight down and in line with torso.
- Top leg rests over and in front of bottom leg.
- Raise shoulder 6 to 8 inches up off ground toward your hip, squeezing your obliques and abdominals.
- Return to ground and repeat.
- Switch sides. Repeat exercise.

PRIME MOVERS: rectus abdominis, obliques, inter-transversari
STABILIZERS: hip flexors, gluteals, and muscles of the thigh

WEIGHT-TRAINING EXERCISES

SQUAT

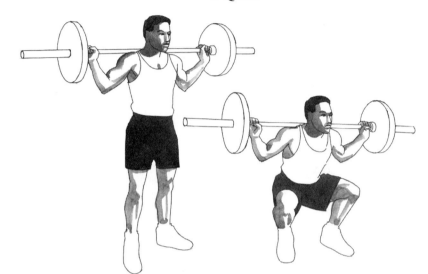

- Use medium to wide overhand grip, raise elbows up in the air to create a muscular shelf for the bar to ride on the posterior deltoids and upper trapezius. Do not place the bar on your neck; it should be below your neck.

- Both feet and hips should be under the bar as you straighten legs to get the bar in and out of the rack.

- Step back and get in a set position: stance should be slightly wider than hips with toes slightly pointed out.

- Your eyes, head, shoulders and chest should all be up with a tight back throughout lift.

- Squat down slowly, leading with the hips, until thighs are parallel to the ground. Do not bounce at the bottom (knees should be in line with toes, don't allow knees to stray inside or outside normal tracking of knee joint); keep weight evenly displaced over feet, do not shift weight forward to toes.

- Raise the bar slowly by straightening out the hips and knees while maintaining correct body position. Keep hips underneath you; don't round back and lean forward on your feet.

- When set is completed, slowly walk the bar back into the rack with both feet and hips underneath the bar. Squat down and lower bar onto the rack.

- Spot from behind, help partner out of rack, squat each rep with him with hands underneath bar or underneath arms near chest. Assist only if necessary by grabbing bar or chest from underneath and having both of you squat the weight up to a safe position. Walk forward and help your partner safely into the rack. Hold bar in and tell your partner he can lower the bar. Adjust not only the bar rack, but the safety bars inside of rack to just below parallel to catch bar if needed.

CLEAN OR HANG PULLS

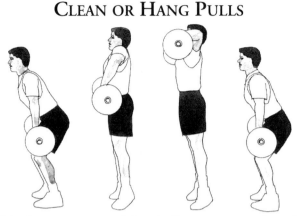

A. Stance = hip width, bar near your shins (refer to power clean beginning position.)
B. Grip: Closed pronated wide grip.
C. Stand up with bar slowly using tight back and legs, arms straight.
D. Cock bar and slide down thighs to power pulling position, just above knees.
E. Initiate pull with legs, hips, and back, keeping arms straight.
F. Shoulders are thrust backward and up.
G. Hips are thrust forward and up.
H. Legs are straightened and extended up onto the toes, before arms begin pulling.
I. The bar stays close to the body.
J. As bar reaches upper chest, there should be a catching effect or bending of the knees to prevent back strain.
K. When lowering the bar, it should be brushed off of the thighs to protect lower back as knees bend upon impact.
L. Return to step D to do more reps; to step C to return bar to the ground.

HANG CLEAN

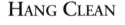

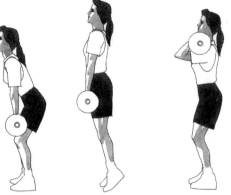

A   Follow above progression to J, except grip should be shoulder width for racking.
B. Body should be lowered to a $1/8$ to $1/4$ squat position before bar starts to descend to prepare for the catch or rack of the bar.
C. Backward rotation of wrists around bar with elbows high and out in front of bar. Bar is carried on shoulders with a bending or cushioning of the legs.
D. Stand up with bar racked. For more reps, go to K and L.

POWER CLEAN AND CLEAN PULL FROM THE GROUND

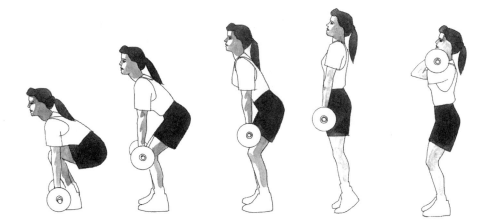

Starting Position:

A. Feet hip width, bar touching shins.

B. Back is flat and tight with shoulders over the bar.

C. Grip the bar with a closed pronated grip (palms facing body).

First Pull:

A. Pull bar from the floor slowly using legs as shoulders remain over the bar with a flat back. Don't jerk bar from floor.

B. Bar stays close to the body with butt down until bar clears the knees.

C. Butt raises a little to prepare for scoop or second pulling phase of lift. Refer to E on Hang Pulls, then following progression of desired lift.

Coaching Points:

A. Coach from the side.

B. Jumping analogy, shoulders over bar for start of second pull, then jump and pull.

C. Drag thumbs along rib cage—high elbows and no looping or reverse curling of bar. This helps in keeping the bar close to your body during the second pull.

D. When racking: Don't catch too deep or wide with stance, keep grip shoulder-width to protect elbows.

E. Always bend knees slightly to protect lower back after the second pull and catch.

LEG PRESS / HIP SLED

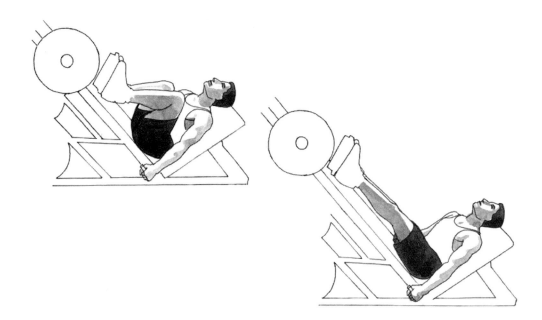

- Lie with back flat on machine and butt touching on pad; use handles to pull butt up against pad and hold this position (especially when legs are at the bottom of the lift).
- Release safety catches and turn them out while raising weight until legs are almost locked out but not completely. Lower weight until legs and thighs have about a 75-90° angle between them. At the bottom of lift, knees should not be forward of toes, if so place feet higher on foot platform or pedals if able. Also butt should be on pad; not off of it with spine rolled up. Keep back flat at all times.
- Slowly push back up almost to full extension but not quite.
- Turn in safety locks and slowly lower weight.

LYING HAMSTRING CURLS
(DOUBLE OR SINGLE LEG)

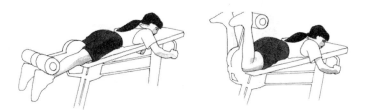

- Lie facedown on machine with pads behind heels.
- Hold on to handles if available.
- Curl legs up; keep flat on the bench until pads touch or almost touch buttocks or back of thigh.
- Return slowly to starting position.
- You may do single leg lying hamstrings curls also.

STEP-UPS
(WITH BARBELL OR DUMBBELL OR BODY WEIGHT ONLY)

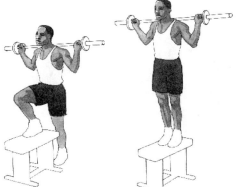

- Start with barbell on shoulders.
- Step up with right leg onto the bench or platform and bring trailing left leg up to standing position.
- Step down under control with right leg first, then left leg to standing position.
- Repeat sequence with opposite leg; alternate legs through set.
- Bench or platform height should have your thigh parallel to the floor when stepping up.
- Dumbbells may be used and held at your sides.

FRONT LUNGE
(DUMBBELL, BARBELL OR BODY WEIGHT ONLY)

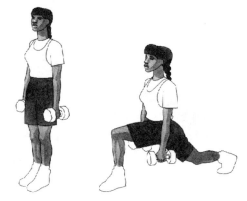

- Start in standing position with dumbbells at your sides.
- Step forward keeping head, shoulders and torso straight up and vertical to the ground.
- Make sure shoulders and hips remain square as you maintain your balance lunging forward until your thigh is parallel to the floor.
- Keep trail leg as straight as possible without touching knee to the ground.
- Push off and step back to starting position.
- Repeat with opposite leg alternating until set is completed.
- You may use your body weight only or a barbell behind your neck like step-ups.

SIDE LUNGE
(DUMBBELL, BARBELL OR BODY WEIGHT ONLY)

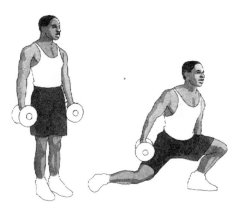

- Start in standing position with dumbbells at your sides.
- Step to the side keeping head, shoulders, and torso upright until thigh is almost parallel to the floor with trailing leg slightly bent.
- Push off and step back to starting position.
- Repeat with opposite leg alternating until set is completed.
- Both dumbbells may also be held in front of you.
- You may use your body weight only or a barbell behind your neck also.

LEG EXTENSIONS

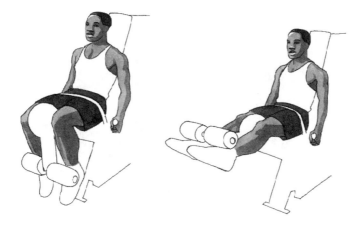

- Sit on machine with pads on shins.
- Knees should be at the edge of seat pad with room to move and should be at least vertical to the floor and maybe a little further back under seat but not too far under seat—that will put extra pressure on the knee joint.
- Use handles and belt if needed.
- Slowly raise legs up to fully extended position, then lower back under control.

STANDING SINGLE LEG HAMSTRING CURLS

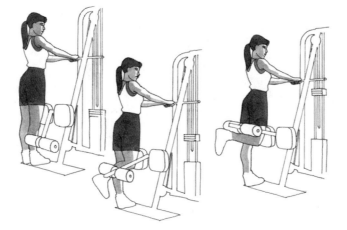

- Start with pad just above your heel and thigh on pad.
- Raise leg upward keeping thigh on pad toward buttocks and touching buttocks if possible at the top.
- Lower under control to the straight leg starting position while keeping thigh on pad.
- Make sure you do both legs; alternating or one leg at a time is OK for reps or sets.

ADDUCTION MACHINE

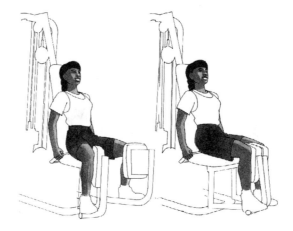

- Start with legs spread and pads just above your knees in a seated position, holding on to the handles.

- Slowly squeeze your knees together until the machine touches; then slowly return to starting position.

- Starting position may be adjustable; start as wide as possible.

- May use single leg low pulley, cables, tubing, etc.

ABDUCTION MACHINE

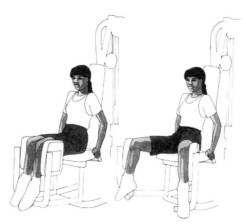

- Start with thighs together, seated with pads just above your knees holding on to the handles.

- Slowly spread your thighs as far as possible against the pads; then return to the starting position.

- May use single leg low pulley, cable or tubing, etc.

STANDING HEEL OR CALF RAISES

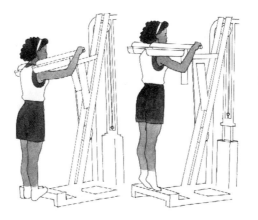

- Stand on platform with pads on your shoulders, straight body, calves stretched with heels down.
- Raise up onto your toes as high as possible and hold for a count; then return to starting position for a count.
- Only joint movements comes from ankle joint.
- May use 2 feet or 1 foot, weight stack or body weight.

BACK EXTENSIONS

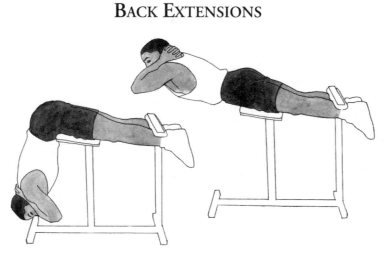

- Place heels under pads and thighs on pad with enough room to bend over.
- Start at bottom with torso in a vertical position and hands behind head.
- Raise torso up until it is parallel to the ground or slightly above the thigh pads.
- Control both raising and lowering phases and don't hyperextend your lower back too much at the top.

STRAIGHT LEG DEAD LIFTS
(BARBELL OR DUMBBELL)

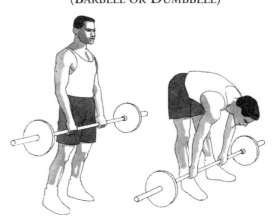

- Start in standing position with a hip width stance and holding bar with straight arms in front of you.
- With knees straight or slightly bent, slowly bend over with straight back lowering the bar along your legs to the top of your feet.
- Return slowly to starting position with a straight back to full standing position.
- Don't bang weight on the floor or bounce at the bottom.
- Do not round back.

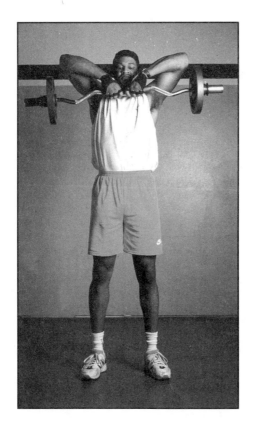

Labradford Smith of the **Sacamento Kings** is performing an upright row with a curl bar.

BARBELL BENCH PRESS

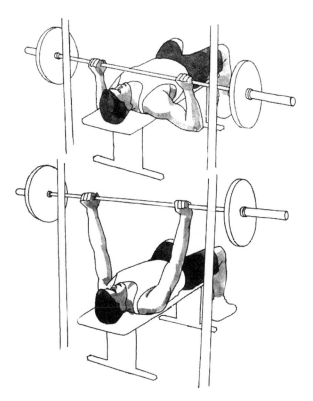

- Lie flat on bench with head, shoulders and buttocks touching surface. Feet are flat and firmly planted on the floor. Maintain this position throughout the lift.

- Grips may vary; in general it should be slightly wider than shoulder width.

- Your head should be not quite underneath the bar, so you may need help out of and back into the rack. This is so the bar won't hit the rack during the exercise.

- The spotter will use an alternating grip and on the count of 3 will help the lifter to the starting exercise position, then release the bar. The spotter will shadow the bar with their hands while not touching the bar unless needed (inside the lifters grip). The spotter will assist with re-racking the bar and let the lifter know when the bar is in the rack.

- When in starting position, slowly lower the bar to the nipple (4"-6" range) on your chest. Grooves vary; this 4"-6" area should fit everyone. Gently touch bar without bouncing and push up to full extension. Use spotter to help you back into rack if needed.

DUMBBELL BENCH PRESS

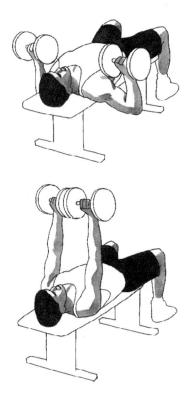

- Once dumbbells are out of rack, stand in front of the bench and sit down on bench, placing dumbbells on your thighs. You may use your thighs to help kick up dumbbell to starting position.

- Lie flat on bench with head, shoulders and buttocks touching surface, feet flat on the floor. Arms are down with dumbbells touching anterior deltoids in a barbell position.

- Slowly press both dumbbells to fully extended position over chest and gently touch them together in between each repetition. Try to press each arm at the same speed and groove as the other arm, controlling the dumbbells is very important.

- Finish with dumbbells over chest; lower them to your thighs as you rock up off the bench. Don't drop dumbbells at the bottom or to the side; this could cause an injury or damage to the equipment.

- Please spot dumbbells from behind by grabbing the wrists and guiding if needed. Dumbbells may float inside, outside, below, or above desired exercise groove.

INCLINE BARBELL BENCH PRESS

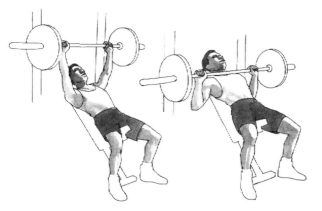

- Lie on bench with head, shoulders and buttocks flat, feet flat on the floor; maintain this position throughout the lift.
- Use medium to wide grip because of different technique grooves on incline and flat bench.
- The spotting will be the same as on the bench press.
- From overhead starting position slowly lower the bar to your upper chest just below your clavicles and gently touch without bouncing. Push-up to full extension. Exercise groove is different and higher on chest and to extended position.

DUMBBELL INCLINE BENCH PRESS

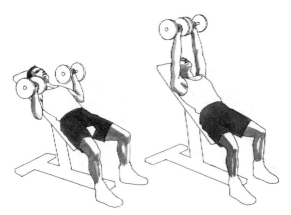

- Stand in front of bench and sit on bench placing dumbbells on your thighs. Kick one knee and dumbbell at a time up to your chest to the starting position touching your anterior deltoids with arms down.
- Head, shoulders and buttocks should be flat on bench with feet firmly on the floor throughout exercise.
- Slowly press both dumbbells to fully extended position gently touching them at the top over your head. Return to starting position when set is complete and place dumbbells on your thighs before getting up off bench.
- Spot by grabbing the wrists and guiding, if needed, from behind.

STANDING MILITARY PRESS

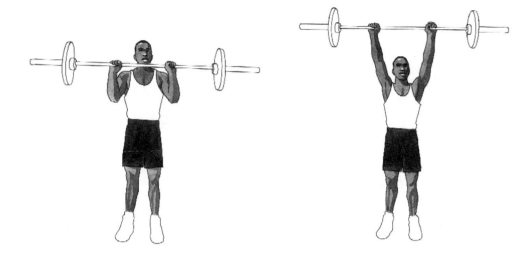

- Follow power clean progression to get to starting point.
- Use shoulder width grip with elbows under bar.
- Slowly press bar to full extension over head (without arching back).
- Lower bar to shoulders under control.
- Spot from behind on bar.

SEATED DUMBBELL SHOULDER PRESS

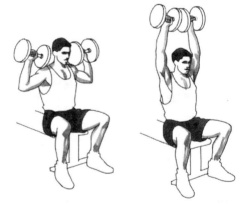

- Seated on the end of the bench with back straight and feet balanced firmly on the floor.
- Either curl up or kick up dumbbells one thigh at a time to starting position just over your outside shoulder.
- Slowly press both dumbbells overhead and gently touch before lowering to starting position.
- Spot by grabbing wrists and guiding if needed from behind.

TRICEP PRESS DOWNS

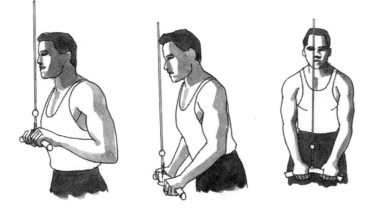

- Grip with palms down approximately 6" to 10" apart.

- Arms and elbows stay fixed and in at your side.

- Hands and bar start up around armpits.

- Press down smoothly moving only your forearms to full extension.

- Return under control to starting position.

LYING TRICEP EXTENSION

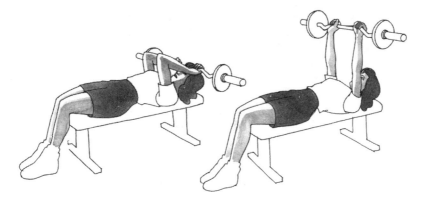

- Lie flat on bench with head, shoulders and buttocks touching surface and feet firmly on the floor; maintain this position throughout lift.

- Use a narrow grip and start with bar extended.

- Slowly lower bar keeping elbows in to the forehead, then extend bar to full lockout over shoulders.

- Forearms only should move, arms should be in a fixed (vertical, straight up and down) position.

BAR DIPS

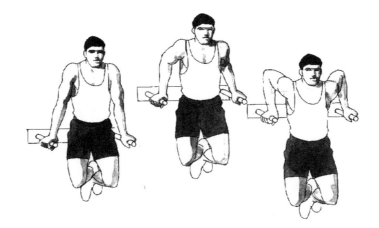

- Start in straight arm locked out position with body erect.

- Slowly lower body under control with elbows in and pointing behind you until shoulders go below elbows. A 90° angle between arm and forearm is minimum depth.

- Press back up to fully extended straight arms.

PUSH-UPS

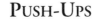

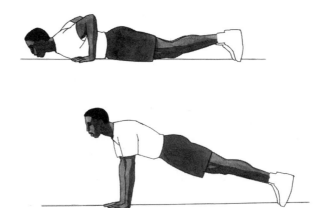

- Hands are slightly wider than shoulders; legs and back are straight while resting up on your toes.

- Keep your body rigid in a straight line; push your body up to full extension; then lower to within 1" of the floor.

- Repeat for desired reps.

PULL-UPS: WIDE GRIP BEHIND THE HEAD

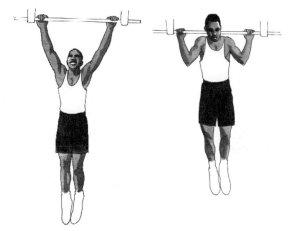

- Hang from the bar with pronated grip and hands wider than shoulders with body and arms straight.

- Pull up until back of neck touches the bar keeping legs fairly straight and without jerking the body.

- Return slowly to starting hanging position with straight arms.

PULL-UPS: MEDIUM GRIP IN FRONT

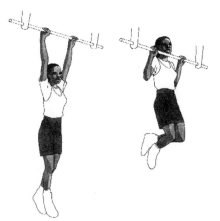

- Hang from bar with pronated grip and hands slightly wider than shoulder width and body and arms hanging straight.

- Pull up until chin is over bar, keeping legs fairly straight and without jerking the body.

- Return slowly to starting position with arms straight.

WIDE GRIP LAT PULLDOWNS BEHIND HEAD

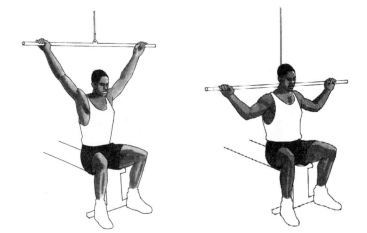

- Sit on bench; put legs underneath thigh pads if available with torso vertical to the floor.

- Make sure arms are straight at the top starting position with hands in a wide pronated position.

- Pull bar straight down slowly without moving torso until it touches the back of the neck; then return under control to straight arm starting position.

NARROW GRIP LAT PULLDOWN IN FRONT

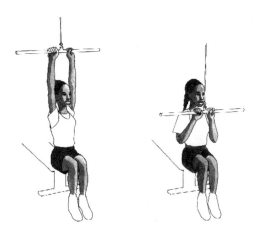

- Sit on bench; put legs underneath thigh pads if available with torso vertical to the floor.

- Make sure arms are straight at the top starting position with a shoulder width pronated grip.

- Pull bar straight down slowly without moving torso to just below your chin; then under control return bar to starting position.

LOW PULLEY SEATED LAT ROW

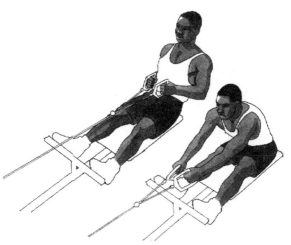

- Seated on pad with legs slightly bent, place feet on the bar, pedals, etc.; with torso in a forward leaning position grab the handles with straight arms.

- Slowly pull back on handles with arms and hands to stomach or low chest position while lower back and torso moves from a forward lean to a slightly backward lean during the pulling phase. Knees remain bent.

- Slowly return to starting position.

DUMBBELL LAT ROW

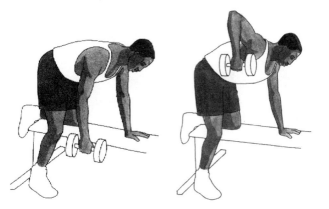

- Place right hand and right knee on the bench with torso parallel to the ground.
- Left arm is straight or hanging with dumbbell; left leg is slightly bent on toes for balance.
- Pull dumbbell up to outside shoulder area with a high elbow at the top of pull and touch the shoulder.
- Don't jerk the weight up; use a steady pull.
- Slowly lower the weight back to starting position.
- Switch arms after set is completed.

LATERAL SHOULDER FLY MACHINE

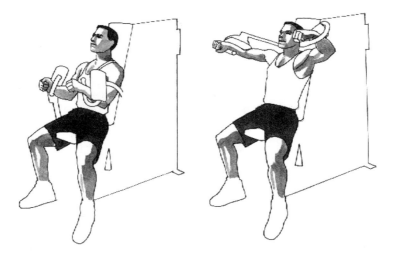

- Sit with back against pad and feet on the ground with pads on forearms.

- Slowly raise forearms and elbows to above shoulder joint and then slowly return to starting position.

DUMBBELL UPRIGHT ROW

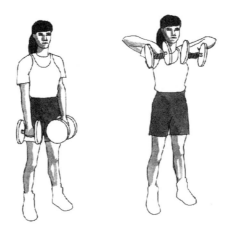

- Standing with arms straight, rest dumbbell against your thighs with thumbs in and facing each other.

- Pull dumbbells straight up the body without swinging them out away from the body to just below the chin with high elbows at the top.

- Knees should be slightly bent.

- Slowly lower dumbbells under control through the same groove to the starting position.

BARBELL UPRIGHT ROW

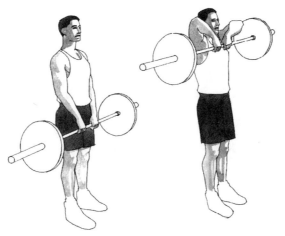

- Stand straight, with the bar resting against thighs, arms straight, hands 4" to 8" apart in a pronated grip.

- Pull barbell straight up the body without swinging it out away from the body to just below the chin with high elbows at the top.

- Knees should be slightly bent.

- Slowly lower the bar in the same groove to original position.

SEATED DUMBBELL LATERAL SHOULDER RAISES

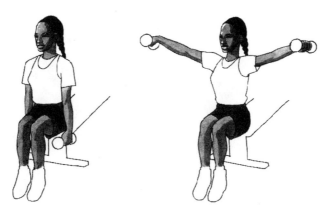

- Sit on the end of a bench with torso vertical to the ground and arms with dumbbells hanging down straight at your sides, feet firmly on the floor.

- Slowly raise dumbbells with knuckles up, elbows slightly bent, slightly above shoulders like a bird's wings. Pause at the top and lower under control to starting position in same groove.

- You may do same exercise standing with knees slightly bent.

SEATED ALTERNATING DUMBBELL CURLS

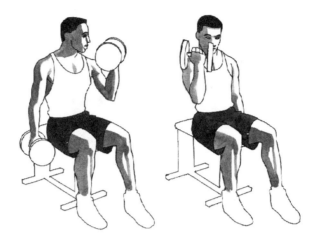

- Sit on end of bench, torso straight, with arms straight at your sides, palms facing in, feet on floor.

- Curl dumbbell until past thigh; then pronate (palm up grip) to finishing position in front of shoulder. Lower under control in same groove to starting position.

- Repeat with other arm alternating reps until set is complete.

- Don't swing weights up; keep elbows in at your sides.

STANDING CURL BAR CURLS

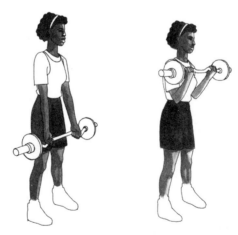

- Assume hip width stance with legs slightly bent, hands on outside angle on curl bar with arms straight and bar resting on thighs.

- Curl bar up keeping elbows in at sides until hands are in front of shoulders at the top.

- Don't swing bar up or let elbows turn out.

- Slowly lower bar in the same groove to starting position.

WEIGHT-TRAINING PROGRAMS

Each weight-training program should be designed with an individual athlete in mind. Each program should address specific strengths, weaknesses, priorities, needs, and target areas. Of course, we can't prescribe individual programs for you because we don't know you. But we can show you three different programs with options that would fit the needs of most every athlete, regardless of sex, age, ability, or experience.

Each of these programs use functional exercises for basketball that will also enhance proper muscle balance as it relates to movement efficiency and injury reduction. Each program has 1 to 3 recovery days in between workouts. Research shows the best recovery time for muscle repair and replenishment to be 48 to 96 hours (depending upon many variables).

BASIC FITNESS PROGRAM

The first program, Basic Fitness, has been designed for the younger or beginning athlete, as a starting point. It works mainly on body-weight-resistance exercises in order to develop muscular strength and endurance. Many of these exercises can be done without weight equipment or weight machines. You may do this program 3 times a week (MON-WED-FRI or TUE-THU-SAT), or 2 times a week (MON & THU or TUE & FRI). You may do 1 to 3 sets of each exercise, starting with one set and progressing to 3 sets as your fitness level dictates.

1. Push-ups: 1-3 sets x maximum repetitions
2. Pull-ups: 1-3 sets x maximum repetitions
3. Bar Dips: 1-3 sets x maximum repetitions
4. Step-ups: 1-3 sets x 10-15 repetitions each leg
5. Lunges   1-3 sets x 10-15 repetitions each leg
6. Back Extensions   1-3 sets x maximum - 20 repetitions
7. Abdominal Crunches   1-3 sets x maximum - 50 repetitions
8. Leg Raises   1-3 sets x maximum - 50 repetitions

THE 3-DAY TOTAL BODY PROGRAM

This program may be used by the beginner, intermediate, or advanced athlete. It was designed for the player who has only 3 days during the week to lift weights.

You may do this program MON-WED-FRI or TUE-THU-SAT. Allow one day recovery in between workouts. Wednesday's program works the same muscle groups as the MON-FRI program, but uses different optional exercises.

You may start on either upper- or lower-body exercises. Whichever you decide, finish that body segment completely before starting the second body segment exercises. This program may take a little longer because of doing the total body each workout. You may speed up the program by super setting 2 exercises at the same time. (Refer to workout card explanation of super setting).

Sets and repetitions are listed in the sample 12-week off-season weight training cycle for this program.

3-DAY TOTAL BODY PROGRAM
MON-WED-FRI OR TUE-THU-SAT

MONDAY AND FRIDAY

1. Bench Press
2. Lat Pull Down
3. Shoulder/Military press
4. Curl Bar Curls
5. Bar Dips
6. Squats/Leg press

7. Power Clean
8. Lying Hamstring Curls
9. Standing Heel Raises
10. Back Extensions
11. Abdominal Crunches

WEDNESDAY

1. Incline Bench Press
2. Lat Row
3. Upright Row/Lateral DB raises
4. Tricep Press Downs
5. Dumbbell Curls
6. Steps-ups + Front and Side Lunges. 2 x each exercises

7. Clean Pull
8. Single Leg Hamstring Curls
9. Single Foot Heel Raises
10. Straight Leg Dead Lift
11. Leg Raises

On Monday and Friday if available, do abduction-adduction exercises.

4-DAY SPLIT PROGRAM

This program may also be used by the beginner, intermediate, or advanced athlete. This design allows a 2- to 3-day recovery time in between the same muscle groups and allows you to focus on one body segment per workout—upper body or lower body. The workouts may be shorter depending on whether you super set and on how many exercises you perform.

The workout days are Monday and Thursday, Tuesday and Friday. You may choose what days (MON, THU, or TUES, FRI) to do either upper-body or lower-body programs.

This workout plan is also forgiving. If you miss a day, you should still have enough open days to get all of your workouts in. This workout is designed to super set the exercises with the same number on the workout cards. These exercises most often use opposing muscle groups or exercises that will not interfere with each other, but will actually enhance each other. Some advantages of super setting include:

1. Faster workouts
2. Proper muscle balance
3. Increased conditioning levels
4. A cleaner neuromuscular signal, recruitment and function
5. Increased blood flow to body segments being exercised

Sets and Repetitions are listed on the Sample 12-Week Off-Season Weight Training Cycle for this program.

4-DAY SPLIT ROUTINE

LOWER BODY: MON AND THU

1. Squat, Hip Sled or Leg Press
1. Lying Hamstring curls

2. Power Cleans or Clean Pulls

3. Step-ups, Lunges or Leg Extensions
3. Single Leg, Seated or Standing Hamstring Curls

4. Side Lunges or Abduction-Adduction Exercises
4. Standing Calves or Heel Raises

5. Back Extensions or Straight Leg Dead Lift
5. Hanging Leg Raises: Straight
                          Bent
                          Sides

UPPER BODY: TUE AND FRI

1. Bench Press: Bar, Dumbbell or Machine
1. Pull-ups or Lat Pull Downs

2. Incline Bench Press: Bar, Dumbbell or Machine
2. Lat Row: Machine, Pulley, Dumbbell or T-Bar

3. Shoulder Press: Bar or Dumbbell, Seated or Standing
3. Upright Row, Lateral DB Raises or Shoulder Fly Machine

4. Bar Dips or Tricep Press Downs
4. Bicep Curls: Seated or Standing, Bar or Dumbbell

5. Abdominal Crunches

SETS AND REPETITIONS? WHAT DO I DO?

There are as many different programs as there are athletes. The age groups that we have targeted are high school and older. If you're younger than high school age, please look at the Glossary listing in the Appendix for Prepubescent Weight Lifting. Young athletes in general should lift lighter weights with higher repetitions (12 to15) per set for safety and health reasons. We have put together a sample 12-week off-season Weight-Training Cycle that will match up with your blank weight-training cards that give you a logical progression for sets or repetitions for all exercises upper and lower body.

This progression is based on research that has been done in the weight-training field in recent years. The chart listed below identifies the 5 major phases of progression for weight-training, the sets and reps for each phase and the volume and intensity for each phase.

THEORETICAL MODEL OF STRENGTH TRAINING
(MODIFIED FOR THIS BOOK)

Phase	Hypertrophy	Basic Strength	Strength & Power	Maintenance	Active Rest
Sets	3 - 4	3 - 4	3 - 4	3	1 - 2
Reps	8 - 12	4 - 6	2 - 3	10 - 8 - 6	15 - 20
Intensity	low	high	high	moderate	low
Volume	high	moderate	low	moderate	high

Does not include warm-up sets; target sets only.

The Hypertrophy Phase is important because it prepares you in two major ways for the higher-intensity phases to come later in the cycle.

1. Hypertrophy is the increase in muscle tissues as a result of specific physiological adaptations to training. Increases in muscle tissue improve your chances of developing strength and power.

2. Your anaerobic capacity or specific endurance related to weight-room exercises and workouts will improve. This will help you in the later phases of the training cycle allowing you to better handle the higher intensities.

The Basic Strength Phase is in between the Hypertrophy phase and the Strength & Power phase. Increases in strength development on all major lifts occur in this phase. You may also notice that the training intensity is high for this phase as increases in both strength and intensity help prepare you for the Strength & Power phase.

The Strength & Power Phase has high intensity and decreases in volume. This aids in the continued strength and power development by lowering the repetitions and focusing on target sets without the fatigue associated with higher-repetition phases.

For the purpose of this book, this could also be called a peaking phase.

The Maintenance Phase is designed to maintain as much of the strength and power achieved in the off-season program as possible throughout the season. For this book the maintenance phase will be the in-season program. There are many different in-season programs depending on many variables; here we will talk about some basic adjustments.

IN-SEASON ADJUSTMENTS

1. Try to get in two weight workouts per body part each in-season week. If you have two days or more before the next game, you may lift heavier, following the suggested 10-8-6 set repetitions for this book. If you have only one day off in between games, you may lift lighter, following the same 10-8-6, or you may do 15-12-10, 3 x10, etc.

2. In-season programs cut back on the number of exercises per body segment, usually using one exercise per muscle group.

3. In-season programs may do the total body each workout with cut-back exercises and fewer potential lifting days.

4. On lighter lifting days, exercise substitutes may take place. (Squats to leg extensions, step-ups or hip sled; cleans to straight leg deads or back extensions; bench press to machine or dumbbell bench.)

5. Depending on game, practice, and travel schedules, there may be time for only one lower body workout a week.

In general, in-season programs should cut back the number of exercises, intensities, and frequency compared to the off-season program. High-risk or certain technique lifts should be adjusted or eliminated in-season as well. These adjustments are made to avoid overtraining between practice, games, workouts, etc.; overtraining may lead to decreased performance or injury.

Listed below is an example of an in-season program with options. The sets and repetitions represent a heavier quality day of the in-season weight workout. Lighter day workout repetitions may be 15-12-10, 3 x10, light 10-8-6, etc.

UPPER BODY

Exercise		Repetition
Chest:	Bench or incline; bar, machine or dumbbell	10-8-6
Back:	Pull-ups, lat pull downs, pull overs or rows	3 x max pullups 10-8-6
Shoulders:	Machine or dumbbell shoulder flies, upright rows bar or dumbbell	3 x 10
Biceps:	Curl bar or dumbbell curls	10-8-6
Triceps:	Tricep press down, tricep extension/press or bar dips	3 x 10
Abdominals:	(See "Abdominal Workout")	4 x 30-50

LOWER BODY

Exercise		Repetition
	Power cleans or clean pulls (may do once a week)	3 x 5
Quadriceps:	Squats, hip sled, leg extensions or step-ups	10-8-6
Hamstrings:	Lying, seated or standing	10-8-6
Groin—inner thigh and lateral hip:	Abduction-adduction machine, pulley or tubing optional or 1 one day a week	2 x 10-15
Lower back:	Straight leg dead lifts or back extension (may substitute for cleans once a week)	2 x 10-15
Abs and hip flexors:	Hanging leg raises: straight, sides, knee-ups	2 x 10-20 each

The **Active Rest Phase** is also called the Post-Season time period in this book. This is the 2 to 8 week time period immediately following the season. The length will vary depending on your situation. During this time the body and mind should recover from the stresses placed on them during the season. Activities should be low in intensity and high in volume to allow the body to recover while still being somewhat active. Two light workouts a week with 1 or 2 sets of 15 to 20 repetitions per exercise is a good parameter; circuit workouts may be used here also. It's a good idea during active rest to do some cross-training in different sports activities as well, but keep the intensity of the activity low for recovery purposes.

12-Week Off-Season Program. The 12-week, off-season cycles match your workout cards, except that they have the number of weeks listed at the top of the page of the prescribed sets and repetitions for each exercise. Certain exercises will have high school repetitions indicated by "H.S." for that exercise. If you're college age or older, you may follow the non-H.S. designated set and repetitions. If you're younger than high-school age, refer to the Scientific Terminology section of the appendix under "Prepubescent Weight-Training" for sets and repetitions.

On the major lifts, squat, leg press, power clean, bench press, incline press, etc., the sets and repetitions prescribed include target sets only. They don't include warm-up sets. (Refer to "Sets" in the Scientific Terminology section).

In target sets, use the heaviest weight possible while maintaining proper technique and performing all of the prescribed repetitions in a set.

The 12-week off-season cycle is your program, please follow all of it the way it was designed for best results in the 3-day and 4-day split programs.

Basic fitness and in-season programs are listed earlier in this chapter and are different from the 12-week off-season cycle program workout cards.

12-WEEK OFF-SEASON CYCLE — UPPER BODY

EXERCISES	3 Weeks	2 Weeks	4 Weeks	1 Week	2 Weeks
1. BENCH PRESS (BAR, DUMBBELL, OR MACHINE)	4 x 10 quality sets	4 x 8 quality sets	4 x 6 quality sets	College 6-4-3-2 H.S. 4 x 6 quality sets	College 5-3-2-2 H.S. 4 x 6 quality sets
1. PRONATED GRIP PULL-UPS / PULL-DOWNS WIDE BEHIND HEAD, SHOULDER WIDTH IN FRONT	4 x maximum or 4 x 10	4 x maximum or 4 x 8 weighted	4 x maximum or 10-8-6-10 weighted	4 x maximum or 10-8-6-10 weighted	4 x maximum or 10-8-6-10 weighted
2. INCLINE BENCH PRESS (BAR, DUMBBELL, OR MACHINE)	4 x 10 quality sets	4 x 8 quality sets	4 x 6 quality sets	College 6-4-3-2 H.S. 4 x 6 quality sets	College 5-3-2-2 H.S. 4 x 6 quality sets
2. SEATED LAT ROW OR DUMBBELL LAT ROW, OR T-BAR	4 x 10	4 x 8	10-8-8-6	10-8-8-6	10-8-8-6
3. MILITARY PRESS OR SHOULDER PUSH PRESS (BAR, DUMBBELL, MACHINE, STANDING OR SEATED)	3 x 10 quality sets	3 x 8 quality sets	10-8-6	10-8-6	10-8-6
3. UPRIGHT ROW, SHRUGS, DUMBBELL RAISES, SHOULDER FLY MACHINE	3 x 10	3 x 10	10-8-8	10-8-8	10-8-10
4. TRICEP EXTENSION / PRESS, BAR DIPS, TRICEP PRESS DOWNS	3-4 x maximum or 3-4 x 10 weighted	3-4 x maximum or 3-4 x 8 weighted	3-4 x maximum or 10-8-6- weighted	3-4 x maximum or 10-8-6 weighted	3-4 x maximum or 10-8-6 weighted
4. BICEP CURLS (BAR OR DUMBBELLS)	3-4 x 10	10-10-8-8	10-8-6-6	10-8-6-6	10-8-6-6
5. ABDOMINAL CRUNCHES STRAIGHT BENT ROTARY	30-40 reps each	30-40 reps each	30-40 reps each	30-40 reps each	30-40 reps each

12-WEEK OFF-SEASON CYCLE — LOWER BODY

EXERCISES	3 Weeks	2 Weeks	4 Weeks	1 Week	2 Weeks
1. SQUATS/LEG PRESS	4 x 10 quality sets	4 x 8 quality sets	4 x 6 quality sets	College 6-4-3-2 H.S. 4 x 6 quality sets	College 5-3-2-2 H.S. 4 x 6 quality sets
1. LYING HAMSTRING CURLS	4 x 10	4 x 10	10-10-8-8	10-8-6-6	10-8-6-6
2. CLEAN PULLS OR POWER CLEANS	8-6-6-6 quality sets	H.S. 8-6-6-6 8-6-6-4 quality sets	H.S. 8-5-5-5 8-5-5-4 quality sets	H.S. 8-5-5-5 6-4-3-2 quality sets	H.S. 8-5-5-5 6-4-3-2 quality sets
3. STEP-UPS, LUNGES OR LEG EXTENSIONS	3 x 10	3 x 10	3 x 10	10-8-6	10-8-6
3. HAMSTRING CURLS (SEATED, SINGLE LEG, OR STANDING)	3 x 10	3 x 10	3 x 10	10-8-8	10-8-6
4. SIDE LUNGE OR ADDUCTORS-ABDUCTORS	2 x 12-15	2 x 12-15	2 x 12-15	2 x 12-15	2 x 12-15
4. 3-WAY STANDING CALVES OR HEEL RAISES	2 x 15-25 each way	2 x 15-25 each way	2 x 15-25 each way	2 x 15-25 each way	2 x 15-25 each way
5. BACK EXTENSIONS OR STRAIGHT LEG DEAD LIFTS	3 x 10-15	3 x 10-15	3 x 10-15	3 x 10-15	3 x 10-15
5. LEG RAISES — Bent	2 x 15-30	2 x 15-30	2 x 15-30	2 x 15-30	2 x 15-30
Straight	2 x 10-15	2 x 10-15	2 x 10-15	2 x 10-15	2 x 10-15
Hanging	2 x 15-25	2 x 15-25	2 x 15-25	2 x 15-25	2 x 15-25

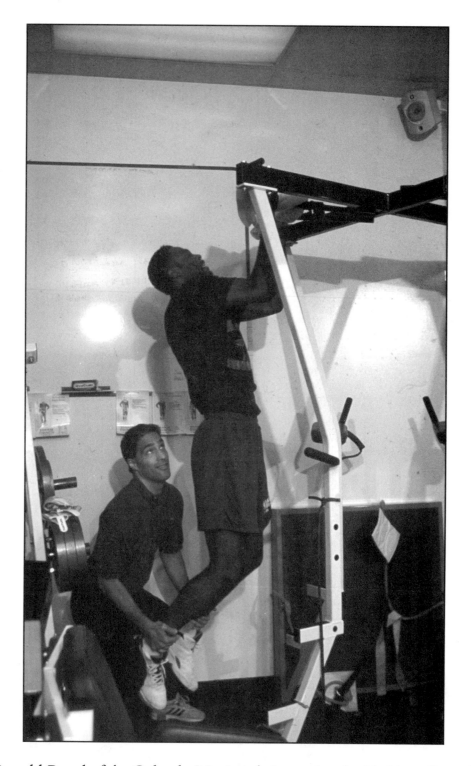

Donald Royal of the **Orlando Magic** is being assisted with his pull-ups by strength and conditioning coach **David Oliver.**

WORKOUT CARDS

The blank workout cards match the 12-week off-season cycle cards. Please make 5-10 copies of the blank workout cards and always keep a blank master for future copying needs. The numbers on the card represent the exercises that should be done together if super setting which was explained earlier in the chapter under the 4-Day Split Program, which we highly recommend for the previously stated reasons.

Do set number 1 of each exercise before progressing to set number 2 of each exercise. Continue this alternating pattern for the prescribed sets or repetitions for each of the exercises super setted throughout the program.

At the top of the card you have a place for your name, and in each daily column you have a place for your body weight, and the date. In the small boxes next to each exercise, list your sets and repetitions.

List the weight first and then your repetitions; the top box is the first set, the second box is the second set , and so on.

Each card/chart has exercise options for most numbers to fit your specific needs: facilities, equipment, favorite exercises, physical limitations, etc.

Bench Press	100 x 15
	135 x 10
	155 x 8
	185 x 6

If you follow the numbers and prescribed sets and repetitions, you'll have a functional program that increases performance and reduces the chances of injury.

WORKOUT CARDS — UPPER BODY

NAME:			
Body Weight:			
Date:			

EXERCISES	Reps:																				

1. BENCH PRESS
(BAR, DUMBBELL OR MACHINE)

1. PRONATED GRIP PULL UPS,
PULL DOWNS (WIDE BEHIND HEAD -
SHOULDER WIDTH IN FRONT

2. INCLINE BENCH PRESS
(BAR, DUMBBELL, OR MACHINE)

2. SEATED LAT ROW OR
DUMBBELL LAT ROW OR T-BAR

3. MILITARY PRESS OR
SHOULDER PUSH PRESS
(BAR OR DUMBBELL, SEATED OR STAND)

3. UPRIGHT ROW, SHRUGS OR
DUMBBELL LATERAL RAISES,
SHOULDER FLY MACHINE

4. TRICEP EXTENSION / PRESS,
BAR DIPS, TRICEP PRESS DOWNS

4. BICEP CURLS
(BAR OR DUMBBELLS)

5. ABDOMINAL CRUNCHES: STRAIGHT
BENT
ROTARY

WORKOUT CARDS — LOWER BODY

NAME:																				
Body Weight:																				
Date:																				
EXERCISES	**Reps:**																			
1. SQUATS/LEG PRESS																				
1. LYING HAMSTRING CURLS																				
2. CLEAN PULLS OR POWER CLEANS																				
3. STEP-UPS, LUNGES OR LEG EXTENSIONS																				
3. HAMSTRING CURLS (SEATED, SINGLE LEG, OR STANDING)																				
4. SIDE LUNGES OR ADDUCTORS-ABDUCTORS 12-15																				
4. HEEL RAISES OR 3-WAY STANDING CALVES 15-25																				
5. BACK EXTENSIONS OR STRAIGHT LEG DEAD LIFTS 10-15																				
BENT 5. LEG RAISES: STRAIGHT HANGING																				

WORKOUT CARDS — BASIC FITNESS PROGRAM

NAME:																
Body Weight:																
Date:																
EXERCISES	**Reps:**															
PUSH-UPS																
PULL-UPS																
BAR DIPS																
STEP-UPS																
LUNGES																
BACK EXTENSIONS																
ABDOMINAL CRUNCHES																
LEG RAISES																

QUESTIONS & ANSWERS

1. Will weight-training throw my shot off?

No. As long as you continue to practice shooting while you train with weights, you will have no difficulty in maintaining the accuracy of your shooting. In fact, you may be able to increase the range of your shooting.

2. Will weight-training make me muscle-bound?

If you perform the exercises through a full range of motion, the flexibility in the specific muscular joints can improve.

3. Isn't it true that weight-training will slow me down?

No. A properly designed weight-training program, along with flexibility, plyometrics, and agility programs, will enhance your speed.

NUTRITION

"You are what you eat." You've probably heard these words a hundred times while you were growing up. Especially when parents or coaches saw you stuffing your face with chips. But it's especially true when it comes to sports. What you eat effects the way you play. If you eat food low in nutritional value, your performance will be less than what it could have been. The foods you consume serve as fuel for your body.

Champion race horses, and even champion racing cars, are fed optimum fuels in high quality diets; only that way can they perform at the height of their capabilities. You can train from sunup to sundown, but if you fail to fuel yourself with the right nutrients, your performance potential will not be reached. In addition, your body will not recover quickly after an exhaustive workout. Your nutritional habits will influence your overall performance.

Many young people think that nutrition is too hard to understand and even harder to put into practice. Of all the factors in the complex equation for improving your athletic performance, nutrition is probably the simplest to do.

You really can "tune up" your performance in a relatively short amount of time by eating better food. Athletic diets vary little from the diets that most people should eat. The main difference is that a young athlete needs more calories to perform better. And, of course, the number of calories that one young athlete may need to perform better differs from another according to such factors as age, sex, body type, and sport type.

CONDITIONING TIP: Nutritional habits influence your performance potential. In your conditioning program, do not forget to eat right.

SCIENTIFIC PRINCIPLES

There are six classes of nutrients:

- water
- carbohydrates
- proteins
- fats
- vitamins
- minerals

WATER

Everyone needs to drink plenty of water. Water is the most critical element in your diet. Under very moderate exercise and weather conditions, you need about two quarts of water per day. Water is necessary for life. Your body needs plenty of water for digestion and food absorption as well as for excreting waste. Water also helps maintain blood plasma levels and is an organ and joint lubricant. You can go a long time without food if necessary; but you cannot survive without water.

Water plays two vital roles when you exercise:

- It regulates your body's temperature, especially the cooling process during workouts.

- It transports both nutrients and by-products into and out of your cells.

Here are some guidelines that you can use for drinking water:

- Drink 6 to 8 glasses of water each day.

- Drink 2 glasses of water 15 minutes before workouts or competition.

- Drink 2 glasses of water beyond thirst requirements after workouts or competitions.

- Drink 1 glass of water every 15 to 30 minutes during workouts or competitions.

- Drink chilled liquids for faster absorption from the stomach into the blood as well as cooling off the body faster.

- Drink 1 glass of water after consuming caffeinated drinks within 12 hours of workouts. Caffeine is a diuretic, which means it will cause dehydration.

Keep in mind that humans do not drink according to an accurate thirst mechanism. Therefore, you will have to train yourself to drink water regularly, especially when you're working out or playing. Keep your body well watered. The experts call it "hydration," and it is an ongoing, life-giving process. We'll discuss sports drinks in another section.

CARBOHYDRATES, FAT, AND PROTEIN

A young athlete should try to eat foods that have an average energy-nutrient distribution as follows:

60-65% Carbohydrate
20-25% Fat
15-20% Protein

All food contains different amounts of calories.

Fat: 9 calories per gram
Carbohydrates: 4 calories per gram
Protein: 4 calories per gram

CONDITIONING TIP: Fat is two times more "calorie-dense" than either proteins or carbohydrates. This means when you read a label that says the food contains 11 grams of fat, it actually has 99 calories!

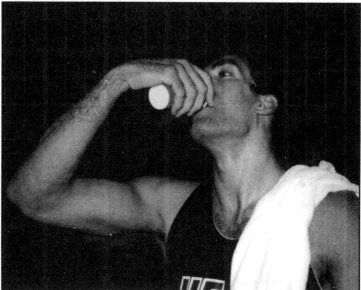

Rony Seikaly of the **Golden State Warriors** knows the importance of staying hydrated during practice.

CARBOHYDRATES

Carbohydrates are composed of sugars and starches. They are divided into two forms: simple and complex.

Simple: some fruits, juices, soft drinks, and sweets
Complex: whole grains, pasta, rice, breads, and vegetables

As the name suggests, a carbohydrate is a substance that's made up of carbon and hydrogen atoms which give a person energy. The most familiar carbohydrate you know is probably sugar. Sugar is the carbohydrate that fuels the body.

Now it may sound at first like the answer to the carbohydrate question would be to drink a lot of soft drinks. Everyone knows that they contain plenty of sugar. However, the sugar contained in soft drinks is a simple sugar that effects your body much differently than complex sugars. Simple sugar provides your body with "quick" energy that will only last briefly. It won't give you enough energy to get you through practice, let alone into the fourth quarter.

Simple sugars, including the things that we call junk food, are not the answer to efficient nutrition. The reason is that they have no nutritional value. Simple sugars are foods that lack nutrients, vitamins, and minerals; they contain "empty calories."

Complex carbohydrates are referred to as complex sugars. These contain nutrients, vitamins, and minerals. Complex carbohydrates include some fruits, vegetables, breads, pasta, and potatoes. Complex carbohydrates are an excellent source of energy.

Your body breaks down complex carbohydrates into glucose. In order to work your muscles effectively, your body requires glucose, which is stored as glycogen in your muscle tissue and liver. Knowing which foods contain simple sugars and which contain complex sugars is the key to fueling your body with the best source of energy.

Since complex carbohydrates are nutritionally dense, you can safely eat larger quantities. This will also give you a more "satisfied" feeling for a longer period of time. As a result, you won't feel like you need to go for that quick sugar pick-me-up.

With regard to the food you eat, your body wants to use carbohydrates as a primary source of fuel. As the length of your athletic activity increases, your body uses fats as energy. And when nothing else is left, it uses protein.

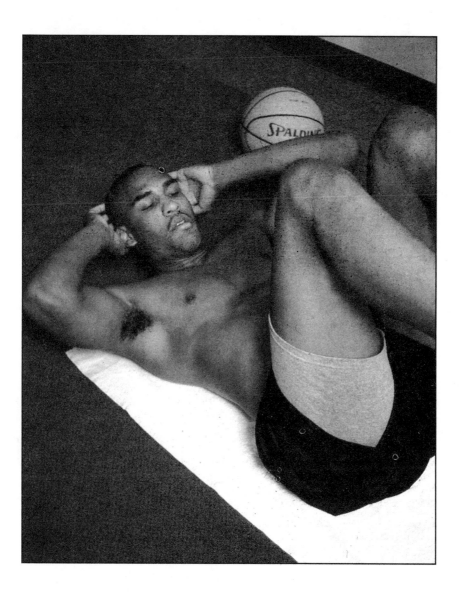

Steve Smith of the **Atlanta Hawks** is working out his abdominals by doing crunches. Crunches strengthen the muscles, they do not get rid of fat. You lower body fat by eating properly and by aerobic conditioning.

PROTEINS

For athletes, muscle tissue is approximately 70 to 75% water, 10 to 25% protein. A diet that is 15 to 20% protein will then meet the needs of nearly all athletes. This is approximately 1 to $1^{1}/2$ grams of protein per kilogram (2.2 pounds) of body weight. A 154 pound teenage athlete needs about 70 grams of protein per day. This requirement could be met with 3 glasses of milk and 2 medium chicken breasts, or the equivalent. Other good sources of protein include beef, pork, fish, eggs, and dairy products.

Protein is the vital substance from which muscles are made. Protein also builds muscles. The subject of protein is often misunderstood; yet it is crucial for healthy nutrition.

By eating large amounts of protein you are not going to get bigger, faster, or stronger. Proper conditioning develops those attributes. Actually protein is a poor source of energy. It is much better to obtain your energy supply from complex carbohydrates.

Your body has certain protein requirements. Once these needs are met extra protein is converted to and stored as fat, or is excreted from your body.

Proteins are actually a combination of smaller units called amino acids. There are 22 known amino acids that are required to support growth and development. Your body can manufacture 13 of them, the other 9 must be provided by your diet. These are considered "essential amino acids." If a food contains all essential amino acids it is considered a complete protein; vegetables are considered incomplete proteins because they lack essential amino acids.

Now no one wants to play a basketball game with an incomplete team. All the necessary players have to be included in order for your team to function effectively. Likewise, for proper nutrition, all of the essential amino acids must be included in your diet.

FATS

It's important to know that fats are a vital part of a well balanced diet. Fats are known as lipids or oils, and are made up of triglycerides. They function to promote the absorption of "fat-soluble" vitamins such as A, D, E, and K. Most of the body's cells use fat in their makeup.

Fat insulates your body and cushions your internal organs. Fat is the only nutrient that remains the same general state throughout the entire digestive process. There is no need to add extra "fatty" foods to your diet. At most we suggest your diet should be composed of 25% fat. The health hazards of high levels of fat accumulation are well-known. Many elite athletes can burn off most of the fat they take in; but we do not suggest using fat as a major source of calories or energy.

The biggest attraction of fat is that food that is high in fat is so flavorful. Meat, ice cream, chocolate, whole milk, cheeses, and many other things that you enjoy contain plenty of fat. Who doesn't like butter on their baked potato? Unfortunately, even margarine with "reduced calories," contains mostly "fat" calories. Fat that is not burned up will be stored as fat.

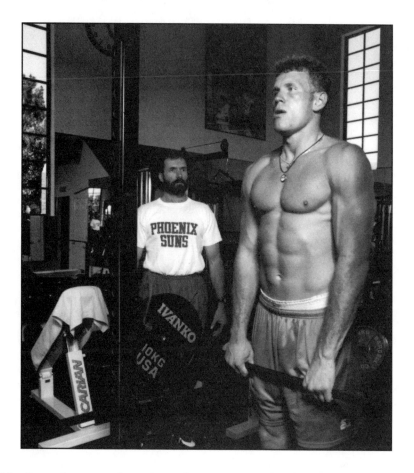

Robin Pound, strength and conditioning coach of the **Phoenix Suns**. is working out **Dan Majerle**. Dan developed his body by working hard and eating right. Nutrition is a big part of Dan's total program.

VITAMINS

Vitamins and minerals are a bit of a mystery to solve in nutrition. Your body needs vitamins (organic compounds) in small quantities. Vitamins help your body perform specific functions essential for proper muscle and nerve functioning, for example Vitamin A helps maintain your vision at night. Vitamins are classified as either fat-soluble (vitamins A, D, E and K) or water soluble (vitamins Bs and C). In addition, vitamins release energy from foods and promote the normal growth of body tissues.

Remember, vitamins are not a source of energy. Some misinformed people take "extra" vitamins without eating in order to receive a boost of energy. Unfortunately, they will only get stomach cramps and pain. Furthermore, water-soluble vitamins aren't stored in the body when you take them in large quantities. As for the fat-soluble vitamins, the excess amount is retained in the body's fat. However, this situation can be dangerous and lead to a condition known as hypervitaminosis; or simply stated, a buildup of toxic levels in the body.

WHAT VITAMINS DO

FAT SOLUBLE VITAMINS

Vitamin A
- Maintains eye and skin health
- Aids resistance to infection

Vitamin D
- Aids absorption of calcium

Vitamin E
- Protects vitamins and essential fatty acids from destruction

Vitamin K
- Needed for blood clotting

WATER SOLUBLE VITAMINS

Vitamin C
- Strengthens body cells
- Promotes healing of wounds and bones
- Increases resistance to infection

Vitamin B$_2$ (Riboflavin)	• Used in energy metabolism
	• Promotes good vision and healthy skin
Niacin	• Used in fat and carbohydrate metabolism
	• Promotes healthy skin, nerves, and digestive tract
Vitamin B$_6$	• Used in protein and fat metabolism
	• Needed for red blood cell formation
Folic Acid	• Used in protein metabolism
	• Promotes red blood cell formation
Vitamin B$_{12}$	• Used in red blood cell development and in maintenance of nerve tissue

MINERALS

Minerals are inorganic substances needed by the body for specific functions. They regulate bodily processes, maintain bodily tissues, and aid metabolism. Calcium, iodine, iron, phosphorous, magnesium, sodium, and potassium are a few of the body's key minerals. They also are called by another name—electrolytes.

Many of these minerals are critical to help your working muscles maintain their contractions over a long period of time.

There are more than 20 mineral elements in the body. Of these, 17 are essential to your diet. Minerals are grouped in two classes; major (macro) minerals are needed in amounts greater than 100 milligrams/day; and trace (micro) minerals, which are only needed in very small amounts.

WHAT MINERALS DO

CALCIUM
- Used to form bones and teeth
- Helps control blood clotting as well as contracting and relaxing muscles

IODINE
- Helps regulate the rate at which your body uses energy

IRON
- An important part of hemoglobin, which carries oxygen throughout your body

MAGNESIUM
- Helps regulate the use of carbohydrates and the production of energy within your cells

PHOSPHORUS
- Combines with calcium to give bones and teeth strength and hardness

POTASSIUM
- Regulates the amount of water in your cells
- Is essential for proper function of the kidneys, heart, and muscles

SODIUM
- Regulates the amount of water in your cells
- Is essential for proper transmission of nerve impulses and contraction of the muscles

ZINC
- Becomes part of several enzymes that affect cell growth and repair
- Is part of insulin, which binds with glucose to carry it through the cell membrane so it can be used as energy

A FINAL WORD ABOUT VITAMINS & MINERALS

If athletes need more vitamins and minerals, they can easily be supplemented in tablet form. The easiest way to do this is to take a children's chewable tablet daily. Chewing insures a greater rate of absorption into your body and helps you control the dosage. Of course, children's supplements are not as potent as adult's. But by using them, you will reduce the amount of waste through excess intake and save a little money.

One comment about salt or sodium. It's everywhere. There's no need to add it to your food. Since salt is an effective preservative, it's put into just about every food you buy, especially in fast-food restaurants.

In conclusion, we want to make a simple point. If you want to be prepared to be your physical best, then learning how to eat is a critical step. Do not become reliant on supplements. First, learn how to eat properly.

The US government now requires food manufactures to list their nutritional makeup, so get in the practice of knowing what you are eating. Learn how to eat nutritionally. In order to make this easy, we encourage you to eat fresh food. The following chart provides some examples of commonly consumed foods.

The remainder of this chapter is designed to help you combine all of this information and make it usable for your daily living.

> "I think a lot of athletes don't realize how important nutrition is to them," says **Don MacLean** of the **Washington Bullets**. "No matter how hard or how much you train, your diet has to be worked on as hard as you train. You can't make gains unless you eat right on a consistent basis."

FASTBREAK

Samples of foods and their nutritional makeup in grams

		Calories	Protein	Carbo-hydrates	Fat
FRUITS:	Apple, 1 medium	80	0	21	0.2
	Banana, 1 medium	121	1	27	0.2
	Orange, 1 medium	60	1	15	0.0
	Grapes, 1/2 cup	35	0	9	0.2
	Peach, 1 medium	35	1	10	0.0
	Cantaloupe, 1/4 medium	29	1	7	0.0
	Pear, 1 medium	101	1	25	0.0
	Strawberry, 1/2 cup	28	1	6	0.0
	Pineapple, 1 large slice	90	0	24	0.0
GRAINS:	White bread, 1 slice	65	2	12	1
	Wheat bread, 1 slice	65	2	12	1
	Spaghetti, 1 cup	155	5	32	1
	Bagel	165	6	28	2
	Corn Flakes, 3/4 cup	72	2	16	0
	Graham crackers, 2	34	1	10	1
	Oatmeal, 1/2 cup	66	2	12	1
VEGETABLES:	Green beans, 1 cup	25	1.6	5.4	0.2
	Corn, 1 cup	135	5.0	34	0.1
	Carrots, 1	30	1.0	7	0.1
	Baked potato, plain	220	5.0	51	0.1
	Tomato, 1/2 medium	22	1.0	5	0.0
	Broccoli, 1 cup	45	5.0	9	0.0

FASTBREAK (CONTINUED)

		Calories	Protein	Carbo-hydrates	Fat
MEAT:	Chicken (roasted), 1/2 breast	140	27	0	3
	Sausage, 1 link	50	2	0	18
	Ground Beef (broiled), 3 oz.	205	20	0	18
	Tuna	135	30	1	0
	Ham (baked), 2 slices	105	10	0	6
DAIRY:	Milk (whole), 1 cup	150	8	11	8
	Milk (2%), 1 cup	120	8	12	5
	Milk (skim), 1 cup	85	8	12	0
	Mozzarella cheese 1 o.z	80	6	1	6
	Swiss cheese 1 oz.	105	8	1	8
	Cream cheese 1 oz.	100	2	1	10
	Butter, 1 tbsp	100	0	0	11
	Margarine, 1 tbsp.	100	0	0	11
	Ice Cream, 1 cup	270	5	32	14
	Frozen Yogurt, 1 cup	200	3	20	3

CONDITIONING TIP: If you want to condition yourself up to peak performance, you must first learn how to eat nutritionally. This is more of a vital step than you may realize.

---

184 • CONDITION THE NBA WAY

GUIDELINES TO NUTRITION

Here is a summary of guidelines that will keep your eating "in bounds":

- Eat low-fat, high-fiber foods.

- Eat more frequent, modestly-sized meals; rather than the typical 3 huge meals a day. A good way to begin this is by increasing your meal frequency to 4 to 6 a day.

- Eat broiled foods instead of fried foods.

- If at first you find it difficult to resist fried foods at least:

    - peel the skin off the chicken, and

    - remove the breading from vegetables.

- Snacks should be fresh fruit and complex carbohydrates instead of sweets or fats.

- Drink plenty of water.

- If you eat sugar or sweets, don't eat them after 6 P.M. Sugar at night suppresses the growth hormone, which is released in your body after strenuous exercise or at night, when you are sleeping. This hormone helps repair your body from daily stresses.

- Alcohol also suppresses the release of the growth hormone. It interferes with the digestion and absorption of nutrients. Remember: Alcohol is a drug, and it harms your body in many ways.

- When you dine at salad bars, eat a rainbow. This means eat a variety of colors (different natural chemical combinations). It will help you obtain the best balance of nutrients from the foods available.

- Ask that your dressings and sauces be placed on the side—that way, you can dip the food in it to reduce your fat intake.

- Be careful eating at fast-food restaurants; they generally serve foods high in fat and sodium content.

- Eat a well-balanced breakfast.

As mentioned above, we believe in the principle of increasing the frequency of meals. This means that even though you'll eat smaller meals each time, you'll eat more often throughout the day. You might soon find yourself enjoying this. Plus it's the best method to fulfill the daily nutritional needs of high performance athletes who need to take in a large amount of calories.

It is also the most efficient method for weight control, if that becomes one of your chosen goals.

For those who have a difficult time gaining weight, you may need to reduce your activity level to give your body time enough to rest and build.

Young athletes especially should make sure they eat large amounts of carbohydrates and make sure they get plenty of protein.

Here's what a sample nutritional schedule might look like. You could use this as a standard from which to create your own nutritional program.

Breakfast	A nutritional shake with fruit and low fat milk, cereal (shredded wheat or similar), toast or bagel. Throughout the morning, drink 2 or 3 glasses of water.
Mid-morning	A single sandwich is sufficient. Or you may like to have yogurt, fruit, bagels, low-fat cookies, Fig Newtons, Graham crackers, Nilla Wafers, or a sports bar. (Watch the sugar content.)
Lunch	Pasta, salad bar, grilled chicken, baked potato, sandwich (tuna, turkey, or chicken), or Chinese food (not fried, and ask for "no MSG"). Resist the temptation to "pig out" at some greasy buffet.
Mid-afternoon	Keep drinking water.
After workout	Repeat either the breakfast or the mid-morning snack. This is a good time to have another nutritional shake.
Dinner	Same approach as lunch.
Evening snack	Have yourself some cookies, cereal, yogurt, or a little fruit.

You may be surprised to see cereal and cookies listed here. There are some good low- to no-fat choices available on your grocer's cookie shelf. However, most of the so-called low-fat variety of chips contain too much fat. Try a few baked tortilla chips with salsa instead. They make a great low-calorie snack!

USDA FOOD PYRAMID GUIDE

The "Four Basic Food Groups" formula used to be the guide for proper nutrition. This formula has been replaced with the "USDA Food Guide Pyramid." This pyramid is more detailed and accurate with the daily servings for the different food groups.

FOOD GUIDE PYRAMID
A GUIDE TO DAILY FOOD CHOICES

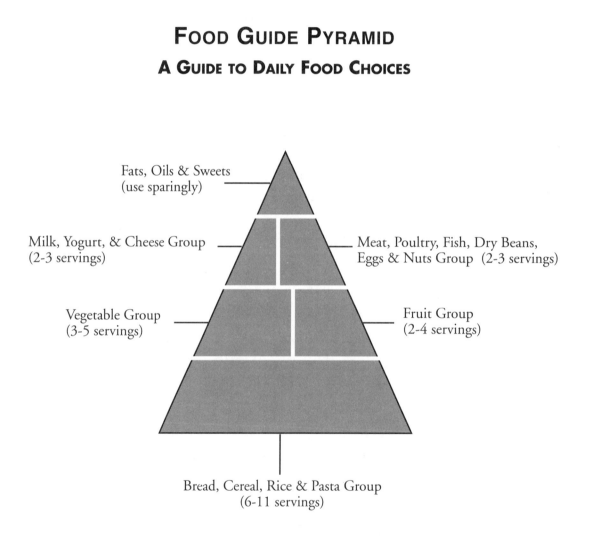

Fats, Oils & Sweets
(use sparingly)

Milk, Yogurt, & Cheese Group
(2-3 servings)

Meat, Poultry, Fish, Dry Beans,
Eggs & Nuts Group (2-3 servings)

Vegetable Group
(3-5 servings)

Fruit Group
(2-4 servings)

Bread, Cereal, Rice & Pasta Group
(6-11 servings)

ENERGY REQUIREMENTS

The average daily energy requirements of young athletes can vary considerably. Caloric intake depends on your body weight, body composition, age, activity level and if you are male or female. The chart below will give you a range of the amount of calories you need to eat each day. If you are training hard, you need to base your calories on the higher numbers.

DAILY ENERGY RECOMMENDATIONS FOR YOUNG MALE AND FEMALE ATHLETES

AGE	CALORIES NEEDED PER POUND OF WEIGHT	
	MALE	FEMALE
11 - 14	24 - 28	20 - 24
15 - 18	18 - 22	16 - 20
19 - 22	18 - 22	16 - 20

CALORIES BURNED PER HOUR DURING VARIOUS EXERCISES

Eating 93	Football (Touch) 476
Bicycling 204	Aerobics (Heavy) 544
Swimming 299	Racquetball 544
Walking 299	Skiing 598
Volleyball 345	Weight-Lifting (Heavy) . .612
Ice Skating 394	Basketball 680
Tennis 414	Running 897
Jogging 476	

PRE-GAME MEAL

The digestion and absorption time of your food is called the gastric emptying rate. Current research indicates that this time can be one to four hours depending on the amounts and types of food in your pre-game meals.

Fats and proteins take approximately three to four hours to digest. Carbohydrates take one to three hours depending on different variables. A pre-game meal should be eaten three to four hours before competition to insure that most of the meal is out of your stomach during competition.

Competition with food in your stomach causes confusion of blood flow between your gastrointestinal tract and your working muscles. This leads to inefficiency in both areas. It may also cause indigestion, cramping, nausea, and vomiting.

Your pre-game meal should follow our nutrition philosophy of high carbohydrate (60-65%), low-fat (20-25%) and the right amount of protein (15-20%). Be sure to drink plenty of water and/or fruit juice throughout the day and with your pre-game meal.

THE DANGER OF EXTREMES

Inside your body are millions, actually billions of cells that comprise your bones, muscles, organs, and glands. As you can imagine, there are many processes going on inside your body at the same time. If any specific area, like muscle growth, receives extra attention while other areas are neglected, then trouble can arise. This is why extremes should be avoided in conditioning as well as in other areas of your life. For instance, if you focus on muscle function and growth, you must quickly learn how that will effect the combined actions of the nervous system and your other internal organs (heart, liver, kidney, digestive system, and brain). All must be cared for in a balanced way to ensure harmony within your body.

Here's an example of one extreme. Let's say a person starts a very high, liquid protein diet in an attempt to increase muscle mass and cut fat. But if the muscles don't receive enough fuel from carbohydrates, they won't be able to perform.

You may recall that protein is not a great energy source. Think of the definition of energy as "the capacity to do work." By not eating properly, you will reduce your capacity to work out.

Furthermore, high protein puts a strain on your kidneys which must filter the by-products out of the blood. Meanwhile, your heart and brain are not receiving enough energy from this high-protein diet. And your nervous system must obtain its energy from carbohydrates. So now you have the problem of protein excess plus deficient carbohydrates and thus insufficient energy.

The same can be said of a very low calorie diet that someone might try for weight loss. Insufficient nutrition and, therefore, energy can lead to a dangerous chain reaction within all the systems of the body.

Conditioning is the major way you have to increase your energy. Some people think that they have to take drastic measures in order to lose or gain weight.

Teenagers have special biological needs that their developing bodies must fulfill. No matter what you think, you cannot deny your body its natural needs without experiencing some negative and possibly dangerous side effects. There are no quick answers, so eat properly and condition wisely.

Here are some questions to ask that may help you avoid harmful extremes.

- Does this program require that I start taking expensive supplements?

- Do I have to start doing things that make me feel weak or tired all the time?

- Is this program built around special timing? In other words, must I learn what foods to eat plus what combinations to take or what pills to ingest at certain hours?

- Is the program I am thinking of using flexible? Can I adjust it to fit my changing schedule?

- Is my program going to be replaced in a couple of months by the new and latest "Euro-fad" diet? (This means then you would have to start everything all over and learn an entirely new program.)

Our goal is to provide you with a long-term, flexible, energy-giving, growth-supporting, and winning program. The thing about our program is that in reality, you can often discover the right choices through your own common sense once you learn the basics.

Fads and Hoaxes

Athletes, like other people, sometimes get caught up in the fads and hoaxes often portrayed to meet special nutritional needs.

Most professional athletes are well aware of the fantastic claims that you see in the magazine ads and the like. After all the glitzy nutritional promises of these products, it may be a relief for you to know that there are no "magical foods or pills" that supposedly give one young athlete an advantage over another.

Education and balance are the keys. It's the surest way to increasing your assets in basketball as well as in other areas of life. It's also the safest way to preventing negative situations from arising due to bad habits.

On the basketball court, a professional athlete learns that his body is his major asset. Just like smart businessmen everywhere, he learns to take excellent care of this asset.

Practice proper nutrition and take care of your major asset—your body.

Fat-Loss Program

When dealing with body weight, we are primarily concerned with your body composition; or, in other words, the amount of lean body mass (muscle) you have in contrast to your total body fat. The major factor here is your percentage of body fat.

If you lose 6 pounds of fat and gain 5 pounds of muscle, the scales will tell you that, after all that hard work, you have lost only one pound. In reality, you have improved your body's composition significantly.

Here are a few things to watch for:

- If you start to notice an increase around your middle, then something is out of line somewhere.

- If you put on weight that you think is good, but you run slower or feel more sluggish, then it is probably unwanted weight.

- If you lose weight that you think is good, but you have a significant drop in strength levels, then you may be losing muscle rather than fat.

If you want to lose or gain weight, plan to do so over a reasonable amount of time (that means weeks or months). Don't try to lose or gain a lot of weight in a short period of time. It may affect your health in negative ways.

NUTRITION AND EXERCISE

Some people believe that being involved in a workout program gives them a blank check to eat as much as they want. This never works.

If you need to drop a few pounds, then please consider doing it sensibly. This means you must patiently work at it on a daily basis. Remember, you are going to be better off both on and off the court by losing at the rate of 3 to 5 pounds per week—tops!

You'll be much healthier, much happier, and you'll make much better decisions (both on and off the court).

HOW TO DISCIPLINE YOURSELF TO LOSE WEIGHT

1. Start by eating sensibly. Eat fewer calories by concentrating on smaller meals and eating complex carbohydrates. Don't skip meals.

2. You need to do at least 20 minutes of daily aerobic (medium intensity) exercise at a pace comfortable enough to complete the conditioning program in order to cut fat.

3. Try cross training. You can ride a cycle, walk, jog, use a stair-climbing machine; or try some interesting combinations like running a mile, then cycling, and so forth. Be creative. Remember, you must increase your activity level in order to lose a significant amount of weight.

When it comes time to eat, follow these nutritional guidelines:

- Low fat
- No simple sugars (the kind found in junk food)
- High carbohydrates
- Medium protein

The mistake many people make in the weight loss game is that they limit their calories but neglect their essentials. For example, some people reduce their protein intake drastically, start losing muscle mass, and then incorrectly assume that they are losing unwanted fat. (Refer to "Dangers of Extremes" earlier in this section for further information.)

As you continue the other parts of the program, be patient with your weight loss. You have to remember that with proper conditioning, it's possible to lose fat and put on muscle. When you proceed in this fashion, you will not notice drastic changes in your body weight. A pound of fat and a pound of muscle weigh the same; but that pound of fat takes up more room than the muscle. Your weight may change very little when you follow this program, but your clothes will fit you much differently.

WEIGHT-GAIN PROGRAM

Gaining weight by building bigger, stronger muscles depends on 3 factors:

> A. Your diet
> B. Weight-training
> C. Heredity

A. YOUR DIET

In order to gain weight you must take in more calories than your body burns. That is, you need to eat more food. You can increase your calories in three ways:

> 1. Eat larger portions at meals
> 2. Eat more meals each day
> 3. Eat snacks between meals

A pound of body weight equals 3,500 calories. If you want to gain weight, you need to eat 3,500 calories more than your body uses. You can gain about 1 pound in a week by eating an extra 500 calories each day.

B. WEIGHT-TRAINING

You must combine your increased caloric intake with a proper weight-training program to gain muscle mass. If you increase your calories and do not exercise, you will get fat. For the proper weight-training program, refer to the Weight-Training chapter.

C. HEREDITY

Genetic potential is the third factor in gaining weight. Some young athletes gain weight at a faster rate than others. If you gain weight slowly, do not get discouraged. Continue with your plan each and every day and good things will happen to you.

You also need to give your body a chance to rest and recover. This will insure that you derive the most benefit from your workouts.

HOW TO USE A POWDER SUPPLEMENT

Use a product with a proper ratio of carbohydrates, proteins, and fats as mentioned earlier in the chapter.

1. BREAKFAST SHAKE:

- 10 to 12 ounces low-fat milk

- 1 cup unsweetened fruit (bananas, peaches, strawberries).

- Suggested amount of powder: use 2 to 3 scoops for approximately 250 to 350 calories. A shake like this can give you a 400 to 500 calorie head start on your day. You can use this after workouts too. Due to the risk of food poisoning, don't add raw eggs for extra protein.

For a really ambitious weight-gaining program, you can add a cup of raw oatmeal to boost you up another 300 calories.

If you're on a weight-loss program, then the shake is a good alternative to skipping a meal. Skipping meals actually slows down your metabolism. That will then compound your weight-loss problem.

If you want to keep your calories in check, you may want to eliminate the fruit from the shake (or use water instead of milk—or try mixing half water and half milk). Use common sense here, and you'll be fine.

2. BEFORE OR AFTER YOUR WORKOUT:

If you use a powder supplement, it should mix easily and thoroughly with water. Drink the supplement 45 to 60 minutes before or after a workout. After is your best choice.

CONDITIONING TIP: A supplement can help you add calories to your diet and assist in your recovery. But don't make supplements the focus of your nutritional program.

QUESTIONS & ANSWERS

I. What about supplements?

Today's supplements include drinks, powders, nutritional bars, and tablets. The questions surrounding them are endless. There are some good ones and bad ones. Realize, there is no one supplement that will turn you into an All-Star. First of all, learn to meet most of your nutritional needs through natural foods. This approach is the fastest way of learning how to eat correctly.

If you decide to take supplements: learn the difference between what they claim to do and what they actually do. For example, good reasons for using a powder supplement or a nutritional bar are: to obtain additional calories; and to obtain additional nutrients, such as vitamins, minerals, carbohydrates, and proteins.

There are plenty of tablets available to take along with the powders. Usually, if you eat well and take a powder supplement, you probably only need to consider taking a multi-vitamin or a mineral tablet. Some research has recently shown that vitamins A, C, and E have important anti-oxidants which help control "free radicals" in the body which can cause internal damage. This knowledge can improve your health and prevent illness; and for athletes it can help speed up recovery.

Think for a minute about what your body wants. Energy is an all-day requirement. You have to supply your own energy by eating properly. If you eat the right foods, then you will gradually provide strengthening vitamins and minerals throughout the day.

The body is a 24-hour-a-day processing operation. Therefore, the large quantity of supplements that you take all must be processed. Now if the surplus is removed, what will you do about your body's needs seven or eight hours later, or after a practice or game? This is why it is so important to learn to eat well. When you eat nutritionally, your body gets a continuous supply of valuable calories, proteins, vitamins, minerals and everything else that it needs.

The point is: if you want to take supplements, they must fit within your daily nutritional requirements for calories, protein, carbohydrates and fat. Before starting, ask a knowledgeable nutritionist, coach or other resource professional.

2. What about steroids?

Steroids are a double-edged sword. They may increase growth and strength, but they can also severely injure the functioning of your internal organs or kill you. In addition, they can change your personality and cause a host of other unpredictable effects to happen inside your body.

Too many athletes have already suffered (and some have died) from using steroids. Use the prevention ideas in this book to support your decisions to "Keep it natural" and "Don't use drugs."

Remember: Your goal is to develop a lifetime nutritional program. You can adjust your program for your competitive years by adding an extra meal or including more calories. What you want to develop is a nutritional schedule and plan that will keep you healthy now, when you become a better athlete and later as you mature into a healthy adult.

3. What is my optimum weight?

Your optimum weight will keep you strong and fast (you don't want to lose quickness), and is easy to carry. The real answer here resides in finding the right percentage of body fat. A high-level male athlete should have right around 6 to 8% or less body fat; a high-level female athlete should have between 12 to 15% body fat. Height/Weight charts are too general—they don't tell you what you need to know. There are times when athletes are overweight based on such charts. If you start getting over 15% body fat for males and 20% body fat for females, then you need to reevaluate your nutritional program.

4. What can I have at half-time?

Keep the fluids going. Watch out for drinks or anything with too much sugar. If you feel hungry, eat only half of something like a sports bar or piece of fruit. It doesn't take much to put sugar into your blood. As with any other part of a nutritional program, get to know your body and how it responds to the things you eat.

Now this is very important: never experiment with some new super-energy formula at half-time. Stick with what you know works for you already.

NUTRITIONAL CONTENTS OF SELECTED FAST FOODS

	Energy (cal)	Protein (g)	Carbo-hydrates (g)	Fat (g)	Sodium (mg)	Chol-esterol (mg)
KENTUCKY FRIED CHICKEN						
ORIGINAL RECIPE						
Wing	181	25	6	12	387	67
Side breast	276	20	10	17	654	96
Center breast	257	26	8	14	532	93
Drumstick	147	14	3	9	269	81
Thigh	278	18	8	19	517	122
EXTRA CRISPY						
Wing	218	11	8	16	437	63
Side breast	354	18	17	24	797	66
Center breast	353	27	14	21	842	93
Drumstick	173	13	6	11	346	65
Thigh	371	20	14	26	766	121
Kentucky Nuggets (1)	46	3	2	3	140	12
Buttermilk biscuit (1)	269	5	32	14	521	1
Mashed potatoes	59	2	12	0.6	228	1
Chicken gravy	59	2	4	4	398	2
Kentucky fries	268	5	33	13	81	2
Corn on the cob	176	5	32	3	21	1
Cole slaw	103	1	12	6	171	4
Potato salad	141	2	13	9	396	11
Baked beans	105	5	18	1	387	1

McDonald's

Egg McMuffin	293	18	28	12	740	299
Hotcakes with butter & syrup	413	8	74	9	640	21
Scrambled eggs	157	12	1	11	290	545
Pork sausage	180	8	0	16	350	48
English muffin with butter	169	5	27	5	270	9
Hashbrowns	131	1	15	7	330	9
Biscuit with sausage	440	13	32	29	1080	49
Biscuit with sausage & egg	529	20	33	35	1250	358
Biscuit with bacon, egg & cheese	449	17	33	27	1230	336
Sausage McMuffin	372	16	27	22	830	64
Sausage McMuffin with egg	451	22	28	27	980	336
Apple Danish	389	6	51	18	370	25
Iced cheese Danish	395	7	42	22	420	47
Cinnamon raison Danish	445	6	57	21	430	34
Raspberry Danish	414	6	62	16	210	26
Hamburger	257	12	30	9	450	37
Cheeseburger	308	15	31	14	750	53
Quarter-pounder	414	23	34	21	660	86
Quarter-pounder with cheese	517	28	35	29	1150	118
Big Mac	562	25	42	32	950	103
Filet-O-Fish	442	14	38	26	1030	50
McD.L.T.	674	28	46	42	1170	112
Chicken McNuggets	288	19	16	16	520	65
French fries, regular	220	3	26	11	110	9
large	312	4	37	16	155	12
Vanilla milk shake	354	10	56	10	170	41

PIZZA HUT
NUTRITIONAL VALUE PER SLICE OF PIZZA

THIN 'N CRISPY:

Standard cheese	340	19	42	11	900	22
Standard pepperoni	370	19	42	15	110	30
Supreme	400	21	44	17	1200	13
Super Supreme	400	21	44	17	1200	13

THICK 'N CHEWY:

Standard cheese	390	24	53	10	800	18
Standard pepperoni	450	25	52	16	900	21
Supreme	480	29	52	18	1000	24
Super Supreme	590	34	55	26	1400	38

FOOD RECORD CHART

After reading this nutrition section, you may be curious about how many calories and grams of carbohydrates, protein, and fat you eat in a day. You can chart this information on the food record chart. If you need more information there are many books that offer complete nutritional make-up of common foods.

Food	Protein	Carbo-hydrates	Fat	Calories

BC POWER RATING™

Now that you've begun the conditioning process by doing drills and exercises in the various chapters, how do you know you're making any headway? To help you chart your progress, we've come up with a BC (Basketball Conditioning) Power Rating. BC Power Rating™ is a new self-test to track your progress. This tool has eight components.

The components which make up the BC Power Rating™ measure power, agility, quickness, strength, muscle endurance, flexibility, and percentage of body fat. As you improve in each of these categories, you'll become a better athlete and a better basketball player. (Before attempting these tests, be sure to properly warm up and stretch out.)

The BC Power Rating™ is a fun way to monitor your improvements and compete with your friends. Once you've attained a 10 in one of the tests, don't get complacent. Continue to work to improve yourself.

VERTICAL JUMP

PURPOSE

The vertical jump is a test that measures explosive power of the lower body.

STANDING REACH

1.   Stand sideways next to a wall with your feet flat on the floor.

2.   Mark the fingertips of your reaching hand with chalk.

3.   Reach with that arm as high as possible and make a chalk mark on the wall.

4.   Tape a yardstick to the wall, with the bottom of the stick resting on the chalk mark and the top of the stick pointing toward the ceiling.

JUMP REACH

1.   Re-chalk your fingertips.

2.   Stand sideways next to the wall and jump as high as possible, tapping the yardstick with your fingertip. (Don't take a step before jumping.)

3.   The difference between the standing reach and the jump reach is your vertical jump.

4.   Jump 3 times and record your best height.

5.   Compare your best jump with the jumps in the "Vertical Jump Power Rating."

VERTICAL JUMP POWER RATING

Females	Males	Rating
≥21"	≥34"	10
20"	32"	9
19"	30"	8
18"	28"	7
17"	26"	6
16"	24"	5
15"	22"	4
14"	20"	3
13"	18"	2
≤12"	≤16"	1

VERTICAL JUMP WORKSHEET
(to be filled in monthly)

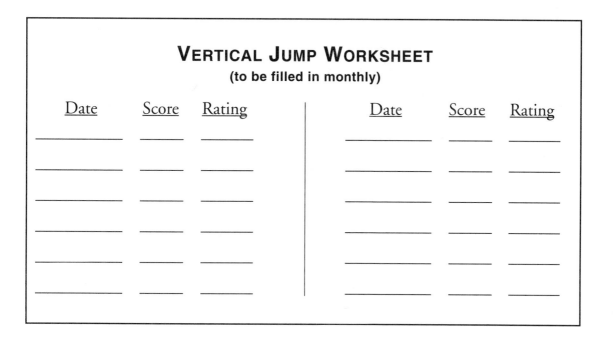

Date	Score	Rating		Date	Score	Rating
_____	_____	_____		_____	_____	_____
_____	_____	_____		_____	_____	_____
_____	_____	_____		_____	_____	_____
_____	_____	_____		_____	_____	_____
_____	_____	_____		_____	_____	_____
_____	_____	_____		_____	_____	_____

20-YARD AGILITY DRILL

PURPOSE

The 20-yard agility drill measures your ability to accelerate, decelerate, and change direction.

PROCEDURE

1. On a flat surface (preferably a gym or possibly a driveway), place a 2-foot piece of tape to mark a center line. Measure 5 yards in both directions from the center line and mark these spots with the tape.

2. Have a coach or friend time you.

3. Straddle the center line with your feet an equal distance from the line and place one hand on the line.

4. On the command "Ready, Go" run toward the line of your choice and touch it with your hand and foot. Change direction and run past the center line to the opposite line and touch it with your hand and foot. Again change direction and run through the center line. This time do not touch the center line with your hand and foot . The drill is over when you cross the center line the second time.

5. Record the best of 3 trials.

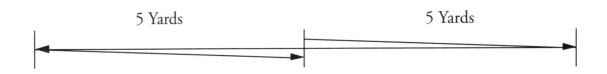

5 Yards   5 Yards

20-YARD AGILITY POWER RATING
TIME (IN SECONDS)

Females	Males	Rating
≤4.5	≤4.0	10
4.8	4.3	9
5.1	4.6	8
5.4	4.9	7
5.7	5.2	6
6.0	5.5	5
6.3	5.8	4
6.6	6.1	3
6.9	6.4	2
≥7.2	≥6.7	1

20-YARD AGILITY DRILL
(to be filled in monthly)

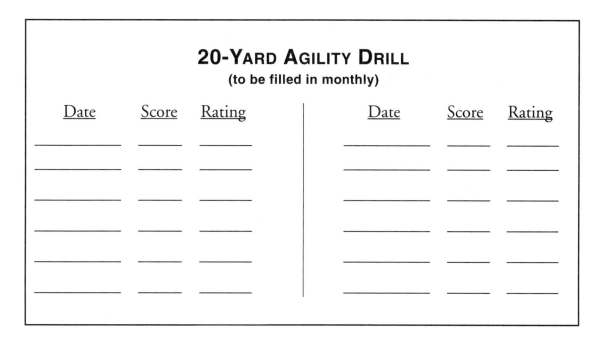

Date	Score	Rating		Date	Score	Rating
___	___	___		___	___	___
___	___	___		___	___	___
___	___	___		___	___	___
___	___	___		___	___	___
___	___	___		___	___	___
___	___	___		___	___	___

300-YARD SHUTTLE

PURPOSE

The 300-yard shuttle is a conditioning test that measures your anaerobic endurance.

PROCEDURE

1. On a flat surface (preferable a gym or track), measure and mark 25 yards.

2. You'll run to the 25-yard mark, touch it with your foot, then turn and run back to the start. Repeat this 6 times without stopping.

3. Rest 5 minutes and repeat the shuttle.

4. Record the average of the 2 times.

25 Yards

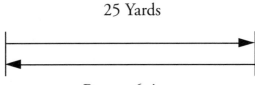

Repeat 6 times

300-YARD SHUTTLE
POWER RATING
TIME (IN SECONDS)

Females	Males	Rating
≤50.9	≤45.9	10
51-52.9	46-47.9	9
53-54.9	48-49.9	8
55-56.9	50-51.9	7
57-58.9	52-53.9	6
59-61.9	54-56.9	5
62-63.9	57-58.9	4
64-65.9	59-60.3	3
66-67.9	61-62.9	2
≥68.0	≥63.0	1

300-YARD SHUTTLE
(to be filled in monthly)

Date	Score	Rating		Date	Score	Rating

PUSH-UPS

PURPOSE

The push-up test measures the muscular strength and endurance in an upper-body pushing movement.

PROCEDURE

1. Assume a proper push-up starting position: straight arms with hands flat on the floor, your thumbs directly below your armpits, and your fingers pointing forward. Your shoulders, back, buttocks, and legs are in a flat, straight position with toes touching the floor.

2. Place a rolled towel (2" high) on the floor directly below your chest.

3. Lower your body under control until your chest touches the towel, and then push your body up until your arms are fully extended.

4. Count the total number of completed repetitions.

5. A repetition isn't counted if:
    - your chest doesn't touch the towel;
    - your body didn't maintain a flat, straight position throughout the movement;
    - arms are not fully extended.

6. The test is over when you can't do a complete a push-up.

PUSH-UPS
POWER RATING
NUMBER OF PUSH-UPS

Females	Males	Rating
≥30	≥60	10
27-29	55-59	9
24-26	50-54	8
21-23	45-49	7
18-20	40-44	6
15-17	35-39	5
12-14	30-34	4
9-11	25-29	3
6-8	20-24	2
≤5	≤19	1

PUSH-UPS
(to be filled in monthly)

Date	Score	Rating		Date	Score	Rating

PULL-UPS

PURPOSE

The pull-up test measures the muscular strength and endurance in an upper-body pulling movement.

PROCEDURE

1. The pull-up bar should be high enough to allow you to hang in a fully extended position without your feet touching the floor.

2. Position your hands on the bar with palms facing away, shoulder-width apart, and the arms in a fully extended hanging position.

3. Pull yourself up until your chin is above the bar and return to a fully extended hanging position.

4. Count the total number of completed repetitions.

5. A repetition isn't counted if:
   - your chin doesn't clear the bar;
   - you fail to fully extend your arms; or
   - your body swings.

6. The test is over when:
   - you fail to complete the upward movement; or
   - you don't begin the upward movement within 5 seconds of completing a repetition.

PULL-UPS
POWER RATING
NUMBER OF PULL-UPS

Females	Males	Rating
≥9	≥16	10
8	14-15	9
7	12-13	8
6	10-11	7
5	8-9	6
4	6-7	5
3	4-5	4
2	3	3
1	2	2
0	≤1	1

PULL-UPS
(to be filled in monthly)

Date	Score	Rating	Date	Score	Rating

SIT-UPS

PURPOSE

The sit-up test measures the muscular strength and endurance of the abdominals and hip flexors.

PROCEDURE

1. Lie on the floor with your knees bent so that your heels are 12 to 18 inches from your buttocks. Interlock your hands with your fingers and place them behind your head.

2. Your partner will hold your feet in position, count your repetitions, and time you for 60 seconds.

3. On command, sit up until your elbows touch your knees, and lay back until your shoulder blades touch the floor. Repeat as many times as possible for 60 seconds.

4. A repetition isn't counted if:

    *   Your elbows don't touch your knees.
    *   Your shoulder blades don't touch the floor.
    *   Your fingers and hands separate, or your hands come over the top of your head.

SIT-UPS
POWER RATING
NUMBER OF SIT-UPS

Females	Males	Rating
≥55	≥60	10
50-54	55-59	9
45-49	50-54	8
40-44	45-49	7
35-39	40-44	6
30-34	35-39	5
25-29	30-34	4
20-24	25-29	3
15-19	20-24	2
≤14	≤19	1

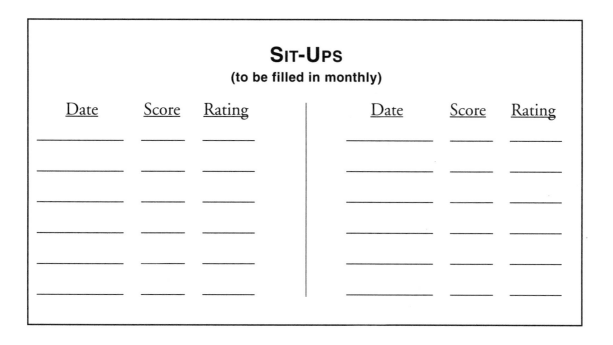

SIT-UPS
(to be filled in monthly)

Date	Score	Rating		Date	Score	Rating
_____	_____	_____		_____	_____	_____
_____	_____	_____		_____	_____	_____
_____	_____	_____		_____	_____	_____
_____	_____	_____		_____	_____	_____
_____	_____	_____		_____	_____	_____
_____	_____	_____		_____	_____	_____

SIT-AND-REACH

PURPOSE

The sit-and-reach is the flexibility test that measures your hamstring and low-back flexibility.

PROCEDURE

1. Sit with your legs extended in front of you and with the bottom of your feet touching the bottom step of a flight of stairs; your feet should be about 6" apart.

2. Set a ruler on the first step so it overhangs in your direction. The inch mark on the ruler that marks the bottom of your feet will be zero for the test. Reaching beyond your feet indicates positive numbers. Not reaching your feet are negative numbers.

3. Keeping your legs straight, bend forward slowly from the waist with your arms outstretched, your hands together, and your palms down.

4. Reach as far as possible with your hands at toe level. Hold for 2 seconds, repeat 3 times, and record your best score.

SIT-AND-REACH
POWER RATING
MEASURED IN INCHES

Females	Males	Rating
≥12	≥10	10
+10	+8	9
+8	+6	8
+6	+4	7
+4	+2	6
+2	0	5
0	-2	4
-2	-4	3
-4	-6	2
≤6	≤8	1

SIT-AND-REACH
(to be filled in monthly)

Date	Score	Rating		Date	Score	Rating
___	___	___		___	___	___
___	___	___		___	___	___
___	___	___		___	___	___
___	___	___		___	___	___
___	___	___		___	___	___
___	___	___		___	___	___

BODY COMPOSITION

We include body composition because it's very important to know your percentage of body fat.

The most effective way to check your body fat is by underwater weighing. It's expensive and requires elaborate equipment and a trained staff.

The easiest way of measuring body composition is to use skin-fold measurements with a caliper. This can be obtained rather easily, but must be done by someone with professional experience.

This professional pinches the skin at 3 to 7 sites on the body and measures the thickness of each fold. He then totals the numbers and uses a chart to calculate your percentage of body fat.

Your Physical Education teacher or a doctor, nurse, or dietician may be able to help you with this procedure. If not, you should see a strength and conditioning coach or fitness trainer.

BODY-COMPOSITION POWER RATING
PERCENTAGE OF BODY FAT

Females	Males	Rating
12.0-13.5	6-7.5	10
13.6-15	7.6-9	9
15.1-16.55	9.1-10.5	8
16.6-18	10.6-12	7
18.1-19.5	12.1-13.5	6
19.6-22	13.6-15	5
22.1-23.5	15.1-16.5	4
23.5-25	16.6-18	3
25.1-26.5	18.1-19.5	2
≥26.6	≥19.6	1

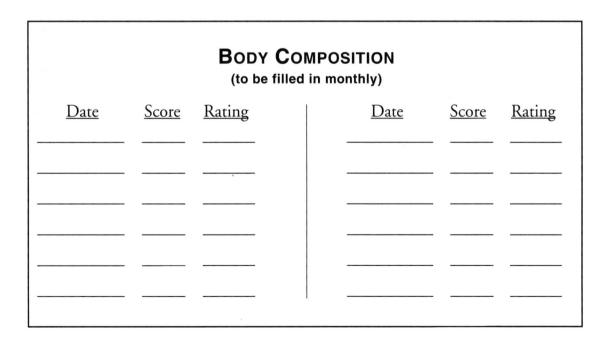

BODY COMPOSITION
(to be filled in monthly)

Date	Score	Rating		Date	Score	Rating
____	____	____		____	____	____
____	____	____		____	____	____
____	____	____		____	____	____
____	____	____		____	____	____
____	____	____		____	____	____
____	____	____		____	____	____

Fill out the BC Power Rating™ chart once a month, and in 12 months' time you'll notice steady progress. Work hard, and don't become discouraged. Be sure to check the age-group averages for your Total BC Power Rating.

AVERAGES BY AGE GROUP

Junior High School (12 to 14 years old)	2 to 4
High School (15 to 17 years old)	4 to 6
College (18 to 21 years old)	6 to 8

Keep up the good work! Have fun sharing your scores with your friends.

BC Power Rating™

TEST	Date ___		Date ___		Date ___		Date ___		Date ___		Date ___		Date ___		Date ___		Date ___	
	Score	Rating	Score	Rating	Score	Rating	Score	Rating	Score	Rating	Score	Rating	Score	Rating	Score	Rating	Score	Rating
Vertical Jump (inches)																		
20-Yard Agility (seconds)																		
300-Yard Shuttle (seconds)																		
Push-Ups (repetitions)																		
Pull-Ups (repetitions)																		
Sit-Ups (repetitions)																		
Sit and Reach (inches)																		
Body Composition (percentages)																		
Total																		
Divide by 8																		
BC Power Rating																		

PUTTING IT ALL TOGETHER

The calendar on the next page shows you how the total program fits together.

On Mondays and Thursdays, you can do your plyometrics and agility training before or after your upper-body weight training. On Tuesdays and Fridays, you should do your strides (conditioning) after your lower-body weight-training. When the sprinting program starts (during week 7) you have 2 choices:

1. You do your sprints on Tuesdays and Fridays before your lower body weight training.

2. You do your sprints on Wednesdays and Saturdays.

Remember, becoming a well-rounded athlete involves a number of components. These components must work together or you may overtrain and decrease your performance. On the other hand, if you neglect any components of the program, you will also experience decreased performance.

This calendar shows a 12-week total program. When you begin this program, the exercises are intended to be low intensity, high volume. The low intensity, high volume phase should be followed by higher intensity, lower volume, with peaking at the end of the program. The calendar is intended for you to use as a daily check system to monitor your total program.

CONDITIONING TIP: Each day, work on your weakest areas first.

OFF-SEASON TOTAL PROGRAM

Month _____   Year _____

Monday	Tuesday	Wednesday	Thursday	Friday	Saturday
Week 1					

Warm up [ ]
Stretch [ ]
Weight train
  upper body [ ]
Plyometrics [ ]
Agility [ ]
Cool Down [ ]
	Warm up [ ]
	Stretch [ ]
	Weight train
	  lower body [ ]
	Conditioning
	  strides [ ]
	Cool Down [ ]
			Warm up [ ]
			Stretch [ ]
			Weight train
			  upper body [ ]
			Plyometrics [ ]
			Agility [ ]
			Cool Down [ ]
				Warm up [ ]
				Stretch [ ]
				Weight train
				  lower body [ ]
				Conditioning
				  strides [ ]
				Cool Down [ ]	

Week 2					

Warm up [ ]
Stretch [ ]
Weight train
  upper body [ ]
Plyometrics [ ]
Agility [ ]
Cool Down [ ]
	Warm up [ ]
	Stretch [ ]
	Weight train
	  lower body [ ]
	Conditioning
	  strides [ ]
	Cool Down [ ]
			Warm up [ ]
			Stretch [ ]
			Weight train
			  upper body [ ]
			Plyometrics [ ]
			Agility [ ]
			Cool Down [ ]
				Warm up [ ]
				Stretch [ ]
				Weight train
				  lower body [ ]
				Conditioning
				  strides [ ]
				Cool Down [ ]	

Week 3					

Warm up [ ]
Stretch [ ]
Weight train
  upper body [ ]
Plyometrics [ ]
Agility [ ]
Cool Down [ ]
	Warm up [ ]
	Stretch [ ]
	Weight train
	  lower body [ ]
	Conditioning
	  strides [ ]
	Cool Down [ ]
			Warm up [ ]
			Stretch [ ]
			Weight train
			  upper body [ ]
			Plyometrics [ ]
			Agility [ ]
			Cool Down [ ]
				Warm up [ ]
				Stretch [ ]
				Weight train
				  lower body [ ]
				Conditioning
				  strides [ ]
				Cool Down [ ]	

Week 4					

Warm up [ ]
Stretch [ ]
Weight train
  upper body [ ]
Plyometrics [ ]
Agility [ ]
Cool Down [ ]
	Warm up [ ]
	Stretch [ ]
	Weight train
	  lower body [ ]
	Conditioning
	  strides [ ]
	Cool Down [ ]
			Warm up [ ]
			Stretch [ ]
			Weight train
			  upper body [ ]
			Plyometrics [ ]
			Agility [ ]
			Cool Down [ ]
				Warm up [ ]
				Stretch [ ]
				Weight train
				  lower body [ ]
				Conditioning
				  strides [ ]
				Cool Down [ ]	

OFF-SEASON TOTAL PROGRAM

Month _____ Year _____

Monday	Tuesday	Wednesday	Thursday	Friday	Saturday
Week 5					
Warm up [ ] Stretch [ ] Weight train upper body [ ] Plyometrics [ ] Agility [ ] Cool Down [ ]	Warm up [ ] Stretch [ ] Weight train lower body [ ] Conditioning strides [ ] Cool Down [ ]		Warm up [ ] Stretch [ ] Weight train upper body [ ] Plyometrics [ ] Agility [ ] Cool Down [ ]	Warm up [ ] Stretch [ ] Weight train lower body [ ] Conditioning strides [ ] Cool Down [ ]	
Week 6					
Warm up [ ] Stretch [ ] Weight train upper body [ ] Plyometrics [ ] Agility [ ] Cool Down [ ]	Warm up [ ] Stretch [ ] Weight train lower body [ ] Conditioning strides [ ] Cool Down [ ]		Warm up [ ] Stretch [ ] Weight train upper body [ ] Plyometrics [ ] Agility [ ] Cool Down [ ]	Warm up [ ] Stretch [ ] Weight train lower body [ ] Conditioning strides [ ] Cool Down [ ]	
Week 7					
Warm up [ ] Stretch [ ] Weight train upper body [ ] Plyometrics [ ] Agility [ ] Cool Down [ ]	Warm up [ ] Stretch [ ] Weight train lower body [ ] Conditioning sprints* [ ] Cool Down [ ]	Sprints* [ ]	Warm up [ ] Stretch [ ] Weight train upper body [ ] Plyometrics [ ] Agility [ ] Cool Down [ ]	Warm up [ ] Stretch [ ] Weight train lower body [ ] Conditioning sprints* [ ] Cool Down [ ]	Sprints* [ ]
Week 8					
Warm up [ ] Stretch [ ] Weight train upper body [ ] Plyometrics [ ] Agility [ ] Cool Down [ ]	Warm up [ ] Stretch [ ] Weight train lower body [ ] Conditioning sprints* [ ] Cool Down [ ]	Sprints* [ ]	Warm up [ ] Stretch [ ] Weight train upper body [ ] Plyometrics [ ] Agility [ ] Cool Down [ ]	Warm up [ ] Stretch [ ] Weight train lower body [ ] Conditioning sprints* [ ] Cool Down [ ]	Sprints* [ ]

* If you do the sprints on Tuesdays and Fridays, they need to be done before weight-training.

OFF-SEASON TOTAL PROGRAM   Month _____   Year _____

	Monday	Tuesday	Wednesday	Thursday	Friday	Saturday
Week 9	Warm up [ ] Stretch [ ] Weight train upper body [ ] Plyometrics [ ] Agility [ ] Cool Down [ ]	Warm up [ ] Stretch [ ] Weight train lower body [ ] Conditioning strides [ ] Cool Down [ ]	Sprints* [ ]	Warm up [ ] Stretch [ ] Weight train upper body [ ] Plyometrics [ ] Agility [ ] Cool Down [ ]	Warm up [ ] Stretch [ ] Weight train lower body [ ] Conditioning strides [ ] Cool Down [ ]	Sprints* [ ]
Week 10	Warm up [ ] Stretch [ ] Weight train upper body [ ] Plyometrics [ ] Agility [ ] Cool Down [ ]	Warm up [ ] Stretch [ ] Weight train lower body [ ] Conditioning strides [ ] Cool Down [ ]	Sprints* [ ]	Warm up [ ] Stretch [ ] Weight train upper body [ ] Plyometrics [ ] Agility [ ] Cool Down [ ]	Warm up [ ] Stretch [ ] Weight train lower body [ ] Conditioning strides [ ] Cool Down [ ]	Sprints* [ ]
Week 11	Warm up [ ] Stretch [ ] Weight train upper body [ ] Plyometrics [ ] Agility [ ] Cool Down [ ]	Warm up [ ] Stretch [ ] Weight train lower body [ ] Conditioning sprints* [ ] Cool Down [ ]	Sprints* [ ]	Warm up [ ] Stretch [ ] Weight train upper body [ ] Plyometrics [ ] Agility [ ] Cool Down [ ]	Warm up [ ] Stretch [ ] Weight train lower body [ ] Conditioning sprints* [ ] Cool Down [ ]	Sprints* [ ]
Week 12	Warm up [ ] Stretch [ ] Weight train upper body [ ] Plyometrics [ ] Agility [ ] Cool Down [ ]	Warm up [ ] Stretch [ ] Weight train lower body [ ] Conditioning sprints* [ ] Cool Down [ ]	Sprints* [ ]	Warm up [ ] Stretch [ ] Weight train upper body [ ] Plyometrics [ ] Agility [ ] Cool Down [ ]	Warm up [ ] Stretch [ ] Weight train lower body [ ] Conditioning sprints* [ ] Cool Down [ ]	Sprints* [ ]

* If you do the sprints on Tuesdays and Fridays, they need to be done before weight-training.

APPENDICES

UPPER BODY	
EXERCISES	**MAJOR MUSCLES WORKED**
Bench press Incline press Bar dips	Pectoralis major Anterior deltoid Triceps bracchii
Lat pull-downs Pull-ups	Latissimus dorsi Rhomboids Teres major Brachioradialis Biceps brachii
Military press Push press	Deltoids Triceps brachii Upper trapezius Supraspinatus Serratus anterior
Seated lat row Dumbell lat row	Latissimus dorsi Rhomboids Teres major Posterior deltoid Biceps brachii Brachioradialis Erector spinae
Lateral dumbell raise	Deltoids Trapezius Supraspinatus
Upright rows	Trapezius Deltoids Biceps brachii Levator scapulae Brachioradialis
Tricep extensions Tricep pressdowns	Tricep brachii Anconeus
Bicep Curls	Bicep brachii Brachialis

LOWER BODY & MIDSECTION	
EXERCISES	MAJOR MUSCLES WORKED
Leg raises Sit-ups (all forms) Crunches involve no hip flexors	Rectus abdominis Obliques (internal and external) Hip Flexors 1. iliopsoas 2. rectus femoris
Straight leg dead lifts back extensions	Erector Spinae 1. spinalis 2. longissimus 3. iliocostalis Hamstrings 1. biceps femoris 2. semimembranosus 3. semitendinosus
Squats Leg press/hip sled Lunges Step-ups	Quadriceps femoris 1. rectus femoris 2. vastus medialis 3. vastus intermedius 4. vastus lateralis Gluteals Erector spinae (squats only)
Leg extensions	Quadriceps femoris
Leg curls: standing or lying	Hamstrings
Abductor machine; (lateral hip) pulley or lying	Abductors 1. tensor fasciae latae 2. gluteus medius 3. gluteus minimus
Adductor machine (inner thigh),pulley, or lying Side lunges	Adductors 1. pectineus 2. gracilis 3. adductor brevis 4. adductor longus 5. adductor magnus
Standing heel raises Seated heel raises,	Calves 1. gastrocnemius 2. soleus

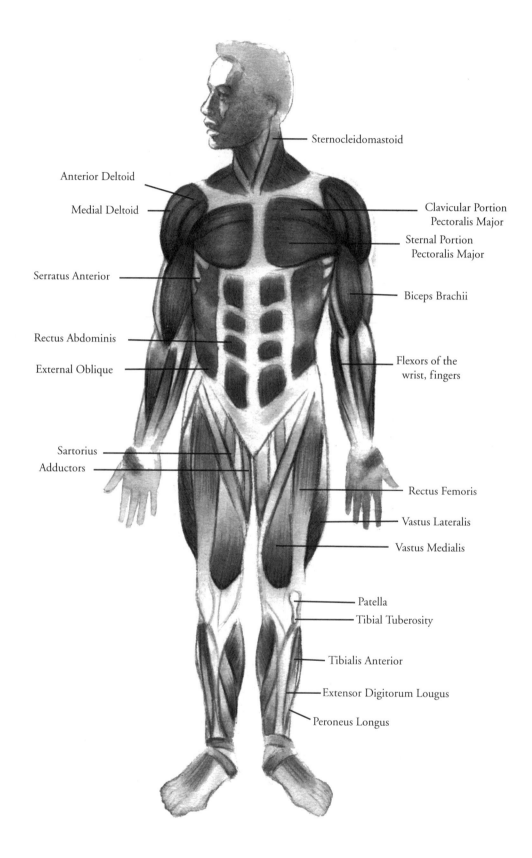

Sternocleidomastoid

Anterior Deltoid

Medial Deltoid

Clavicular Portion
Pectoralis Major

Sternal Portion
Pectoralis Major

Serratus Anterior

Biceps Brachii

Rectus Abdominis

External Oblique

Flexors of the
wrist, fingers

Sartorius

Adductors

Rectus Femoris

Vastus Lateralis

Vastus Medialis

Patella

Tibial Tuberosity

Tibialis Anterior

Extensor Digitorum Lougus

Peroneus Longus

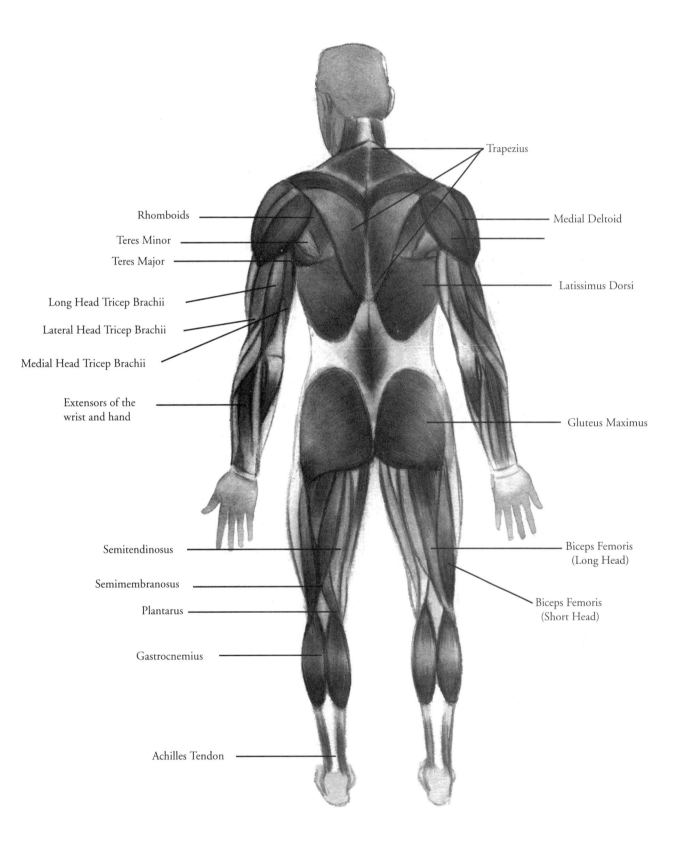

Trapezius

Rhomboids

Medial Deltoid

Teres Minor

Teres Major

Latissimus Dorsi

Long Head Tricep Brachii

Lateral Head Tricep Brachii

Medial Head Tricep Brachii

Extensors of the
wrist and hand

Gluteus Maximus

Semitendinosus

Biceps Femoris
(Long Head)

Semimembranosus

Plantarus

Biceps Femoris
(Short Head)

Gastrocnemius

Achilles Tendon

GLOSSARY

Agonist (prime mover): the muscles primarily responsible for performing the exercise

Antagonist: the muscle or group of muscles that are opposing the prime mover muscle or muscle group

Body-building: the sport in which the body is judged according to various posing positions displaying muscular development, size, balance, and definition

Circuit-training: type of resistance training that is time-controlled with a specific exercise order; the work period and the rest period must be completed in a specific amount of time; this type of training typically incorporates higher repetitions with shorter rest periods

Duration: the amount of time allotted for each rep, set or workout

Eccentric phase: action of the muscle lengthening during its contraction. Eccentric phase as its applies to plyometrics is the *loading* phase of the drill

Fast-twitch fibers: the type of white (light) muscle tissue that is utilized during explosive movements for strength, power, speed

Frequency: how many times (per day, week, etc.) you work out

Golgi Tendon Organ: receptors located where the muscle "fuses" with the tendon (e.g., musculo-tendonous junction). The Golgi tendon organ provides very precise information concerning the tension of the muscle and serves as a protective mechanism to prevent the tendon from rupture as a result of a forceful contraction. The Golgi Tendon initiates an immediate relaxation of the muscle because of too much tension to prevent injury

Hypertrophy: the enlargement of muscle-fiber types as a result of specific training adaptations

In-season: the term applies to strength training performed throughout the competitive schedule when games are being played

Intensity: the effort level exerted while performing an exercise; the intensity of a workout can be changed by changing the exercise order, increasing or decreasing the number of exercises, repetitions, weight, or rest periods

Major muscle groups: the following groups of muscles are considered the major muscle groups of the body: chest, shoulders, back, hips, and thighs

Muscle balance: training opposing muscle groups with the same intensity in order to prevent injury and enhance performance

Muscle movements and contractions

    Isotonic/concentric contraction: refers to the shortening of a muscle during an exercise; for example, the raising of the bar during a bicep curl which shortens the biceps muscle

    Eccentric contraction: refers to the lengthening of a muscle during an exercise; for example, the lowering of the bar during a bicep curl, which lengthens the bicep muscle

    Isokinetic: the speed of movement remains constant no matter how intense the contraction; this type of movement is the result of work on resistance machines that use pistons, shocks, and cylinders

    Isometric: when both ends of a muscle are fixed and no joint movement occurs; physiological work is being done, but not physical work

Muscular endurance: the ability to perform movements over an extended period of time

Muscle Spindle/Stretch Receptors: Located in among, and parallel to the muscle fibers are small spindle shaped mechanisms which sense the rate and length of a stretched muscle.

Off-season: the term applies to strength training performed in the non-competitive season. Twelve (12) weeks prior to pre-season is the standard used in this book

Overload: the term applies to a phase of training that goes beyond the initial output level; overloading the training level by increasing the intensity or duration of an exercise; see Intensity

Overtraining: break-down in the recovery process that may be attributed to mental attitude, lack of sleep or rest, improper eating habits, and over-use of the body

Post-season: the time immediately after the season (2 to 8 weeks); usually called "active rest"

Power: power can be measured by calculating the formula; force times distance divided by time

Power-lifting: weight-lifting in which the sum (1 rep maximum) of three separate weight-training lifts—squat, bench, and deadlift—are totaled

Prepubescent weight training: training associated with young athletes before puberty. The repetitions to perform for each exercise should range between 12 to 15 and 2 to 3 sets in order to reduce the potential risk of injury

Pre-season: the time from the first practice until the first game

Progression: the phase of training in which the intensity of a workout is increased

Range of motion: refers to the specific range of motion suggested while performing an exercise

Repetition: the fully completed movement of the exercise

Set: each time an exercise is performed for a given number of repetitions

> **Warm-up sets:** sets performed to prevent injury and increase the temperature of the muscles and surrounding tissues

> **Target sets:** the quality, hard-working, high intensity sets that follow warm-up sets; each exercise should consist of at least one to two target sets

Stabilizer: usually a non-moving isometric contraction stabilizing one body part so that another body part, usually involving the prime mover, has something to pull against in order to create the movement; for example, in leg lifts, the abdominal muscles are stabilized while the hip flexors are the prime movers

Stretch Reflex: The stretch or myotatic reflex results in the reflex contraction of a muscle after that muscle has been stretched rapidly. When a muscle is rapidly stretched, as occurs during the eccentric or loading phase of a plyometric drill, impulses are discharged by the muscle spindles resulting in a reflex contraction of the stretched muscle. An example of the stretch reflex is the knee jerk test. When the patellar ligament is tapped, the muscle spindles located in the quadriceps femoris send a message to the spine which in turn sends a message back to the "quads" instructing them to contract

Super-setting: performing two or more exercises one after the other before a rest period is taken; a super-set can be performed with exercises for opposing muscle groups, for the same muscle group, or for non-associated muscle groups

Synergist/Assistance Muscle: aids the prime mover with the movement

Total-body joint exercise: movements, are explosive in nature, that involve the ankle, knee, hip, and shoulder joints

Volume: the total number of repetitions performed in a given workout

Warm-up,general: usually uses large muscle groups and non-specific movements to bring out desired physiological changes

Warm-up, specific: duplicates the exact movement or exercise to be performed with very light weight and high repetitions

Weight-lifting: the type of weight-training incorporating the Olympic lifts: the clean and jerk and the snatch

REFERENCES

Alter, Michael J. *Sport Stretch,* Leisure Press, 1990.

American Dairy Council, *Power Food Handout,* 1993.

Baechle, T. "Essentials of Strength Training and Conditioning," *NSCA and Human Kinetics,* 1994.

Briggs, G. and Calloway, D. *Nutrition and Physical Fitness,* 11th Edition, Holt Rinehart, Winston, 1984.

Clark, Nancy. *Nancy Clark's Sports Nutrition Guidebook,* Champaign, IL: Leisure Press, 1990.

Fox, E. L. and Matthews, D. K. *Physiological Basis of Physical Education and Athletics,* 3rd Edition, Chicago: Saunders College Pub., 1981.

Guyton, A. *Textbook of Medical Physiology,* 7th Edition, W. B. Saunders, 1986.

Hickson, J. F. *Nutrition in Exercise and Sport,* Boca Raton, FL: CRC Press, 1989.

Knortz, Karen, M.S., R.P.T., A.T., C. and Ringel C., R.P.T., "Flexibility Techniques," *NSCA Journal,* Volume 7, Number 2, 1985.

McAtee, Robert E. *Facilitated Stretching.* Human Kinetics Publishing, 1993.

Siff, Mel C., Ph.D. "As a System of Physical Conditioning," *National Strength and Conditioning Association Journal,* Vol 13, Number 4, 1991.

Stone, Michael and O'Bryant, H. *Weight Training: A Scientific Approach,* Bellweather Press, Minneapolis: Burgess, 1987.

ABOUT THE AUTHORS

All of the authors of *CONDITION THE NBA WAY* are members of the National Basketball Conditioning Coaches Association (NBCCA). For more information about the NBCCA, contact:

National Basketball Conditioning Coaches Association
2665 South Bayshore, Suite 202
Coconut Grove, FL 33133
(305-859-7787)

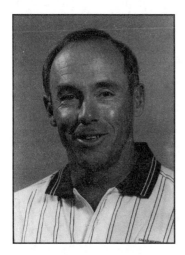

AL BIANCANI — Strength and Conditioning Coach for the **Sacramento Kings**. Previously, Al was the head track and field coach at California State University at Stanislaus. He was also assistant track and field coach at California State University at Sacramento, where he received his undergraduate and master's degree in physical education. Al received his doctorate in physical education from Utah State University. He was chapter coordinator and writer for the Speed chapter.

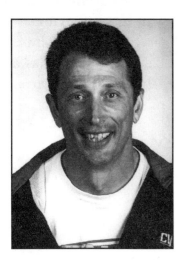

SOL BRANDYS — Strength and Conditioning Coach for the **Minnesota Timberwolves**. Prior to this position, Sol worked as a consultant for the University of Minnesota Athletic Department. He has a Bachelor's Degree in Physical Education from University of Minnesota. He is on the board of directors of the NBCCA and was the chapter coordinator and writer for the Conditioning chapter, as well as a member of the editorial review board.

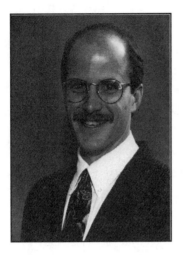

GREG BRITTENHAM — Strength and Conditioning Coach for the **New York Knicks**. Previously, Greg was an associate director for the Center for Athletic Development at the National Institute for Fitness and Sport in Indianapolis. Greg has a B.A. Degree in Physical Education from the University of Nebraska at Kearney and a Master's Degree in Sport Science from Indiana University. Greg was the chapter coordinator and writer for the Plyometrics chapter.

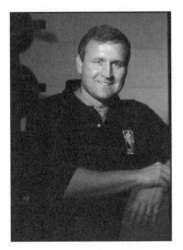

BILL FORAN — Strength and Conditioning Coach for the **Miami Heat**. Before joining the Heat, Bill was the Head Strength and Conditioning Coach for the University of Miami and Washington State University. He has a B.S. in Physical Education and Health Education from Central Michigan University, and a Master's Degree in Exercise Physiology from Michigan State University. Bill is Co-founder and President of the NBCCA. He was the project coordinator for this book, as well as a member of the editorial review board.

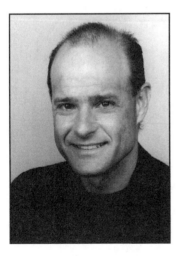

MARK GRABOW — Strength and Conditioning Coach for the **Golden State Warriors**. Previously, Mark worked with Stanford University's men's tennis and women's and men's basketball teams. He has a B.A. in Psychology and Education from American University. He was chapter coordinator and writer for the Agility chapter.

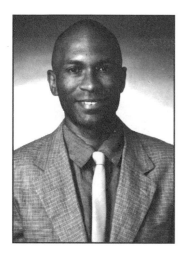

ROGER HINDS — Strength and Conditioning Coach and Assistant Athletic Trainer for the **Atlanta Hawks**. Prior to working for the Hawks, Roger was the Athletic Trainer at St. Francis College in Brooklyn. He also served as the Director of Sports Medicine at the College of Charleston in South Carolina. He has a Bachelor's Degree in Physical Education from Brooklyn College, and a Master's in Physical Education from Indiana State University. Roger was a writer for the Nutrition chapter.

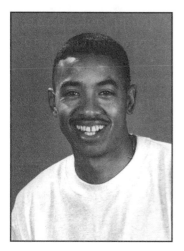

CARL HORNE — Strength and Conditioning Coach for the **Los Angeles Clippers**. Prior to this position Carl worked at the Los Angeles Sports Medicine Clinic. He has a Bachelor's Degree in Physical Education and Dance from University of Nebraska. He was a writer for the Warming Up, Stretching, and Cooling Down chapter.

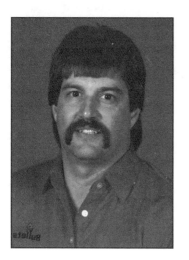

DENNIS HOUSEHOLDER — Strength and Conditioning Coach for the **Washington Bullet**s. Prior to this, Dennis was a high school football coach in Maryland. He has a Bachelor's Degree in Physical Education from Sheppard College in West Virginia. He was a writer in the Weight-Training chapter.

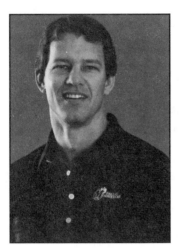

BOB KING — Strength and Conditioning Coach for the **Dallas Mavericks**. He is also currently Defensive Coordinator and Head Track Coach at Trinity Christian Academy. He also serves as an Assistant Strength and Conditioning Coach for the Dallas Cowboys. Bob received a B.A. Degree from Texas Tech. Bob is a co-founder of the NBCCA and is on the board of directors. He is the chapter coordinator and a writer for the Nutrition chapter, as well as a member of the editorial review board.

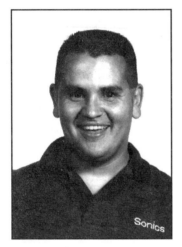

BOB MEDINA — Strength and Conditioning Coach for the **Seattle Supersonics**. Before joining Seattle, Bob was the assistant Strength and Conditioning Coach at the University of Nevada at Las Vegas, where he earned a Bachelor's Degree in Athletic Training. He is a writer for the Conditioning chapter.

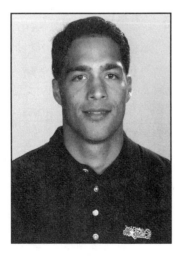

DAVID OLIVER — Strength and Conditioning Coach and Assistant Trainer for the **Orlando Magic**. Previously, David worked at the Orlando Sports Medicine Center and with the Orlando Predators of the Arena Football League. He has a Bachelor's Degree in Exercise Physiology from the University of Wisconsin. David was the chapter coordinator and a writer for the Warming Up, Stretching, and Cooling Down chapter.

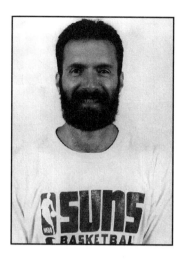

ROBIN POUND — Strength and Conditioning Coach for the **Phoenix Suns**. Before joining the Suns, Robin was the Head Strength and Conditioning Coach for University of California at Berkeley, and Assistant Strength and Conditioning Coach at the University of Oregon. He has a Bachelor's Degree in Physical Education and a Master's Degree in Exercise Physiology and Anatomy from the University of Oregon. He is a co-founder of the NBCCA and on the board of directors. He was the chapter coordinator and writer for the Weight-Training chapter and was on the editorial review board.

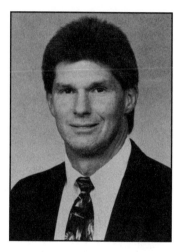

CHIP SIGMOND — Strength and Conditioning Coach for the **Charlotte Hornets**. Prior to this he was the Head Strength and Conditioning Coach at Appalachian State University and Assistant Strength and Conditioning Coach at the University of North Carolina. He has a Bachelor's Degree in Physical Education from Appalachian State University. He was a writer for the Conditioning chapter.

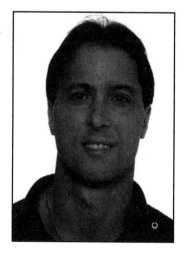

MICK SMITH — Strength and Conditioning Coach for the **Portland Trailblazers**. Prior to working with the Trailblazers, Mick was the Assistant Strength and Conditioning Coach for the University of Miami. He also served as an Olympic Weight Lifting Coach in Saudi Arabia. He has a Bachelor's Degree in Physical Education and Health Education and a Master's Degree in Exercise Science from the University of Nebraska. He was a writer for the Weight Training chapter.